REVERSING CHRONIC DISEASES NATURALLY

A Comprehensive Guide to Natural Healing

Pharm. Fatima I.Abdulkadir

Published in Nigeria:fatiabch@gmail.com

This book is designed to provide information and guidance for individuals seeking to reverse chronic diseases through lifestyle changes and natural therapies. The contents of this book are based on the latest scientific research and the author's personal experiences working with patients to reverse chronic diseases. The information provided in this book is not intended to replace the advice of a qualified healthcare provider. Readers should consult their healthcare provider before implementing any changes to their diet, exercise routine, or medical treatment.

The case studies and success stories featured in this book are based on real-life experiences and have been used with the permission of the individuals involved. Any resemblance to actual persons, living or dead, or actual events is purely coincidental.

The publisher and author are not responsible for any adverse effects or consequences resulting from the use of the information presented in this book. Readers are solely responsible for their own health and well-being.

Are you tired of relying on medications to manage chronic diseases? Do you want to take control of your health and live a happier, healthier life? Look no further than Reversing Chronic Diseases Naturally: A Comprehensive Guide to Natural Healing.

The book thoroughly explores chronic diseases, their causes, and their impact on your health. It offers a holistic approach to reversing chronic diseases through lifestyle changes, natural therapies, and collaboration with healthcare providers.

Discover the power of nutrition, exercise, stress management, sleep, and environmental factors in promoting natural healing. Learn about natural therapies like herbs, acupuncture, meditation, and home remedies and how to choose the right ones for your needs.

In addition, the book provides practical advice on finding healthcare providers who support natural healing and how to communicate with them effectively. You will also find case studies and success stories from real-life individuals who have reversed chronic diseases using natural healing methods.

Do not let chronic diseases control your life. Take charge of your health with Reversing Chronic Diseases Naturally: A Comprehensive Guide to Natural Healing.

Pharm. Fatima I. Abdulkadir

CONTENTS

PHAM FATIMA I. ABDULKADIR

I: INTRODUCTION

A. Overview of Chronic Diseases

Chronic diseases are long-lasting medical conditions typically involving slow progression and persistent symptoms. They are a global health concern and are the leading cause of death and disability. Some of the most common chronic diseases include:

1. Cardiovascular disease: This includes conditions that affect the heart and blood vessels; such as coronary artery disease, heart attacks, and stroke.

2. Diabetes: The body cannot regulate blood sugar levels properly in this condition.

3. Cancer: This group of diseases is characterized by the uncontrolled growth of abnormal cells in the body.

4. Respiratory diseases: These include conditions such as chronic obstructive pulmonary disease (COPD) and asthma.

5. Arthritis: This is a group of diseases that affects the joints and surrounding tissues, causing pain and inflammation.

6. Kidney disease: The kidneys cannot effectively filter waste and excess fluid from the bloodstream in this condition.

7. Neurological diseases include conditions such as Alzheimer's

disease, Parkinson's disease, and multiple sclerosis.

Chronic diseases often develop over many years, making early detection and prevention key to avoiding their negative impact on health. Some of the factors that contribute to the development of chronic diseases include:

i. **Genetics:** Some chronic diseases have a genetic component, meaning they may run in families. For example, genetic mutations that increase the risk of developing certain types of cancer may be inherited.

ii. **Lifestyle factors:** Unhealthy habits, such as a sedentary lifestyle, poor diet, and smoking, can increase the risk of developing chronic diseases.

iii. **Environmental factors:** Exposure to certain chemicals, pollutants, and other environmental toxins can increase the risk of developing chronic diseases.

iv. **Medical conditions:** Certain conditions, such as high blood pressure and cholesterol, increase the risk of developing chronic diseases.

Chronic diseases can significantly impact a person's health and quality of life. For example, cardiovascular disease can lead to heart attacks and strokes. At the same time, diabetes can cause nerve damage, kidney disease, and vision loss. Chronic conditions can also lead to decreased mobility, increased disability, and decreased life expectancy.

Effective management of chronic diseases requires a comprehensive approach that involves lifestyle changes, regular medical care, and appropriate medications. This may include dietary changes, increased physical activity, stress management techniques, natural remedies, and alternative therapies.

Working closely with a healthcare provider to develop a personalized plan for managing chronic diseases is imperative.

With the right approach, many chronic diseases can be prevented, controlled, or even reversed, allowing individuals to live longer, healthier lives.

B. Importance of Reversing Chronic Diseases

Reversing chronic diseases is essential for maintaining good health and improving quality of life. Chronic diseases are long-term conditions that can cause serious health problems and limit a person's ability to carry out daily activities. They include conditions such as heart disease, stroke, diabetes, cancer, and arthritis, to mention a few. Reversing these diseases can forestall the situation's progression and reduce the risk of complications and disability.

Reversing chronic diseases can also lower healthcare costs as these conditions are often expensive to treat and manage. By reversing a chronic illness, individuals can reduce their dependence on medication and improve their overall health and well-being. This can also lead to reduced hospitalization and the need for medical procedures, further lowering healthcare costs.

Reversing chronic diseases improves mental health and enhances the overall quality of life. By reducing a chronic condition's physical and psychological strain, individuals can feel empowered and more confident in managing their health. This can also improve their relationships, increase participation in physical and social activities, and lead to a happier, more fulfilling life.

Other points to consider include:

- **Improved physical function:** Reversing chronic diseases can improve physical function and increase mobility, allowing individuals to carry out daily activities efficiently and independently.
- **Better management of symptoms:** By reversing chronic diseases, individuals can better manage symptoms and

reduce pain and discomfort associated with the condition. This can lead to a more active lifestyle and better overall well-being.

- **Better cardiovascular health:** Reversing chronic diseases such as heart disease and stroke can help improve cardiovascular health and reduce the risk of heart attacks and strokes.
- **Reduced risk of comorbidities:** Chronic diseases often lead to other health problems, known as comorbidities. Individuals can reduce their risk of developing these secondary conditions by reversing the underlying condition.
- **Improved mental health:** Chronic diseases can cause anxiety and depression, further impacting physical health negatively. By reversing chronic diseases, individuals can improve their mental health and reduce the negative impact of stress on their physical health.
- **Better sleep:** Reversing chronic diseases can improve sleep quality and reduce the risk of sleep-related health problems.
- **Increased lifespan:** By reversing chronic diseases, individuals can improve their overall health and increase their lifespan, allowing them to enjoy a longer, more fulfilling life.

In conclusion, reversing chronic diseases is crucial in improving health outcomes and quality of life. By addressing the root causes of these conditions, individuals can reduce the impact of chronic diseases on their health and well-being and live a healthier, happier life.

C. The Approach to Reversing Chronic Diseases

Reversing chronic diseases is a complex process that requires a holistic approach, ranging from lifestyle changes to medical treatments. Here are some of the best practices that can help manage or reverse chronic diseases:

- **Healthy diet:** Adopting a diet rich in whole foods, fruits & vegetables, lean proteins, and healthy fats can help reduce inflammation and improve overall health.
- **Regular physical activity:** Regular physical activity, such as walking, cycling, or swimming, can help improve cardiovascular health and prevent chronic diseases.
- **Stress management:** Chronic stress can worsen symptoms of many chronic diseases. It is, therefore, essential to find healthy ways to manage stress, such as yoga, meditation, or deep breathing exercises.
- **Avoiding harmful substances:** Quitting smoking, reducing alcohol consumption, and avoiding exposure to toxins can help prevent or reverse chronic diseases.
- **Medications:** Depending on the chronic disease, a doctor may prescribe medication to manage symptoms and prevent further damage.
- **Monitoring and managing medical conditions:** Regular check-ups with a doctor and ongoing monitoring of medical conditions, such as blood pressure and blood sugar levels, can help prevent chronic diseases from worsening.
- **Collaboration with healthcare team:** Working with healthcare providers, including a doctor, pharmacist, dietitian, and physical therapist, can help you develop a personalized approach to managing and reversing chronic diseases.
- **Sleep:** Getting enough quality sleep is essential for overall health and can help reduce the risk of developing chronic diseases.
- **Supplements:** In some cases, supplements such as Omega-3 fatty acids, Vitamin D, and probiotics may be beneficial for managing chronic diseases. However,

   talking to a doctor before starting any new supplement regimen is essential.

- **Mind-body therapies:** Techniques such as mindfulness, acupuncture, and massage can help reduce stress and improve overall health, benefiting people with chronic diseases.
- **Social support:** A solid support network, including friends, family, and support groups, can help provide emotional and practical support and benefit people with chronic diseases.
- **Clinical trials:** Participating in clinical trials can give people with chronic diseases access to new treatments that are not yet widely available.
- **Lifestyle changes:** Making lifestyle changes, such as reducing screen time and incorporating more physical activity into daily life can help reduce the risk of developing chronic diseases.

Remember, the best approach to reversing chronic diseases will depend on the specific condition and the individual, so working with a doctor to develop a personalized plan is essential. It takes time and effort.

D. Benefits of Reversing Chronic Diseases?

Anyone who is suffering from a chronic disease can benefit from reversing it. Reversing a chronic illness can improve the quality of life and reduce the risk of future health problems. Chronic diseases, such as type 2 diabetes, heart disease, and certain types of cancer, can be caused by lifestyle factors, such as unhealthy diet, lack of physical activity, and smoking. These can be prevented or reversed by positively changing one's lifestyle. This includes maintaining a healthy diet, exercising regularly, quitting smoking, and managing stress. Working with a healthcare provider to develop an individualized plan for managing and reversing chronic disease is essential.

Other benefits of reversing chronic diseases are:

Lower healthcare costs: Treating chronic diseases can be expensive, and reversing the disease can reduce the need for ongoing medical care and medication.

Improved mental health: Chronic diseases can affect mental health and lead to feelings of depression and anxiety. Reversing the condition can improve self-esteem and overall well-being.

Increased lifespan: Chronic diseases can significantly shorten lifespan, but reversing the disorder can help people live longer, healthier lives.

Enhanced physical functioning: Chronic diseases can limit physical ability and reduce mobility. Reversing the disease can help improve physical functioning and increase energy levels.

Improve sleep: Chronic diseases can cause discomfort and pain, leading to sleep problems. Reversing the disease can improve sleep quality and promote restful sleep.

It is important to note that reversing chronic diseases is a long-term process that requires commitment and consistency. However, the benefits of reversing chronic diseases make the effort well worth it.

E. Overcoming challenges associated with reversing chronic diseases

Reversing chronic diseases can be challenging, but it is not impossible. The following are some of the common challenges and ways to overcome them:

a)   **Lifestyle changes:** Chronic diseases often result from unhealthy lifestyle habits such as poor diet, lack of physical activity, and smoking. Changing these habits can be difficult, especially if they have become ingrained. Overcoming this challenge requires a strong commitment and support from family and friends and the development of new, healthy habits.

b)   **Medication side effects:** Many chronic diseases are managed with medication, but these drugs can have unpleasant side effects. Overcoming this challenge requires a close partnership with your pharmacist to find the right balance between managing the disease and avoiding side effects.

c)   **Compliance:** Taking medications and making lifestyle changes as prescribed is essential to reversing chronic diseases. However, sticking to a treatment plan can be difficult, especially if it involves multiple medications or a strict diet. Overcoming this challenge requires a strong commitment and a clear understanding of the benefits of following the plan.

d)   **Cost:** Chronic diseases can be expensive to manage, and the cost of medications, treatments, and dietary changes can quickly become humongous. Overcoming this challenge may require exploring options for financial assistance, such as insurance, government programs, or patient assistance programs offered by pharmaceutical companies.

e)   **Emotional impact:** Chronic diseases can take an emotional toll, leading to feelings of anxiety, depression, or a sense of hopelessness. Overcoming this challenge requires addressing emotional and physical health and seeking support from family, friends, or mental health professionals.

f)   **Limited access to healthcare:** Access to quality healthcare can be challenging, especially for rural or underserved communities. Overcoming this challenge may involve:
   - Seeking out community health clinics.
   - Telemedicine options.
   - Working with advocacy organizations to improve access to healthcare services.

g)   **Chronic pain:** Chronic diseases such as arthritis, fibromyalgia, and others can cause chronic pain. This pain can be challenging to manage and can impact daily activities and quality of life.

Overcoming this challenge requires a comprehensive approach that may include pain management medications, physical therapy, and alternative therapies such as acupuncture or massage.

h)   **Cognitive changes:** Some chronic diseases, such as Alzheimer's or Parkinson's, can cause cognitive changes that impact memory, decision-making, and communication. Overcoming this challenge requires seeking out support and resources for managing cognitive changes, such as cognitive rehabilitation or speech therapy.

i)   **Social isolation:** Chronic diseases can lead to social isolation, which can exacerbate the physical and emotional effects of the disease. Overcoming this challenge requires connecting with support groups, community organizations, or online resources to stay connected and build a supportive network.

j)   **Treatment adherence:** Following a treatment plan can be difficult, especially if the plan involves multiple medications or a strict diet. Overcoming this challenge requires regular communication with your healthcare provider, tracking progress, and seeking support from family and friends.

By addressing these challenges and seeking out support and resources, people with chronic diseases can work towards reversing their condition and improving their overall health and well-being.

II:UNDERSTANDING CHRONIC DISEASES

A. Chronic Diseases Explained

Chronic diseases are long-lasting conditions that persist for a prolonged period, often for a person's entire life. They are usually characterized by slow progression and can have a significant impact on a person's quality of life. Examples of chronic diseases include cardiovascular diseases (such as heart disease and stroke), diabetes, cancer, chronic obstructive pulmonary disease (COPD), osteoarthritis, and Alzheimer's disease. Chronic diseases often result from a combination of genetic, environmental, and lifestyle factors. They can be managed through treatments such as medications, lifestyle changes, medical procedures or a combination of any of them.

Chronic diseases can have far-reaching consequences beyond just physical health. They can also have a significant impact on a person's mental health, relationships, and overall ability to participate in daily activities. Additionally, they often lead to a cycle of worsening symptoms, increased medical treatments, and decreased mobility, which can have a notable impact on a person's quality of life. Chronic diseases account for the majority of healthcare spends and disability worldwide, posing a significant burden on the healthcare system and the economy.

With proper management and treatment, many chronic diseases can be effectively managed, and their impact minimized. Lifestyle changes such as a healthy diet, regular physical activity, and quitting smoking can help prevent the development of some chronic diseases, and slow their progression. Additionally, it is possible to manage many of them through a combination of medications, therapies, and medical procedures, allowing those who suffer from them to lead full and productive lives.

B. Common Chronic Diseases

Chronic diseases are long-term conditions that often progress slowly and can be managed in the long term. Some of the most common chronic diseases include:

1. Cardiovascular disease: This includes conditions that affect the heart and blood vessels, such as hypertension, coronary artery disease, and heart failure.

2. Diabetes: This condition affects the way the body processes glucose (blood sugar) and can lead to high blood sugar levels.

3. Chronic respiratory disease: This includes conditions such as asthma, chronic obstructive pulmonary disease (COPD), and bronchitis.

4. Cancer: This is a group of diseases characterized by the uncontrolled growth and spread of abnormal cells.

5. Arthritis: This group of conditions affects the joints and can cause pain, stiffness, and inflammation.

6. Chronic kidney disease: The kidneys in this condition are unable to function properly, leading to the buildup of waste products in the blood.

7. Depression: A mood disorder that can cause persistent feelings of sadness, hopelessness, and loss of interest in activities.

8. Osteoporosis: In osteoporosis, the bones become weak and brittle, making them more susceptible to fractures.

9. Alzheimer's disease and other dementias: These conditions affect the brain and can cause memory loss, confusion, and other cognitive problems.

10. Obesity: This is a condition characterized by excess body weight and can increase the risk of other chronic diseases such as cardiovascular disease and diabetes.

11. Parkinson's disease: This neurological disorder affects movement and can cause tremors, stiffness, and difficulty with balance and coordination.

12. Autoimmune diseases: In these conditions, such as rheumatoid arthritis, lupus, and multiple sclerosis, the immune system attacks the body's tissues.

13. Gastrointestinal disorders: These include conditions such as irritable bowel syndrome (IBS), inflammatory bowel disease (IBD), and gastro esophageal reflux disease (GERD).

14. HIV/AIDS: This is a viral infection. It attacks the immune system, leading to a range of health problems.

15. Thyroid disease: This includes conditions such as hypothyroidism and hyperthyroidism, which can affect the body's metabolism and cause a range of symptoms.

It is noteworthy to mention that there are many other chronic diseases beyond these examples, and the prevalence of different diseases can vary depending on factors such as geography, age, and lifestyle.

C. Causes of Chronic Diseases

The causes of chronic diseases are complex, multifactorial and often involve a combination of genetic, environmental, and lifestyle factors. Here are some of the critical factors that contribute to the development of chronic diseases:

- **Lifestyle factors:** Certain lifestyle factors, such as poor diet, lack of physical activity, and tobacco use, can increase the risk of developing chronic diseases.
- **Environmental factors:** Exposure to pollutants, toxins, and other environmental factors can also contribute to the development of chronic diseases.
- **Aging:** As we age, our risk of developing chronic diseases increases due to the gradual decline in our bodily functions.
- **Infections:** Certain infections, such as hepatitis B and C, HIV, and human papilloma virus (HPV), can increase the risk of chronic diseases such as liver cancer, cervical cancer, and AIDS.
- **Chronic inflammation:** Chronic inflammation is like a constant, low-level alarm in your body. It's when your body's defense system stays active for a long time, even when there's no immediate threat. This can lead to health problems over time. Chronic inflammation is believed to contribute to the development of many chronic diseases, including heart disease, diabetes, and cancer.
- **Unhealthy weight:** Obesity and overweight are key risk factors for several chronic diseases, including heart disease, diabetes, and certain cancers.
- **Mental ill health:** Chronic stress, anxiety, depression, and other mental health issues can increase the risk of chronic diseases, such as heart disease, diabetes, and autoimmune disorders.
- **Occupational hazards:** Exposure to certain chemicals and materials in the workplace can increase the risk of developing chronic diseases such as lung disease, cancer, and musculoskeletal disorders.
- **Socioeconomic factors:** Poverty, limited access to healthcare, and lack of education can increase the risk of chronic diseases. They also contribute to disparities in health outcomes.

- **Genetics and epigenetics:** Our genes and the way they are expressed (epigenetics) can influence our risk of developing chronic diseases. For example, some people may be genetically predisposed to conditions like heart disease or cancer. Some specific genetic mutations increase the risk of developing certain chronic disease conditions.
- **Autoimmune disorders:** Autoimmune disorders occur when the body's immune system attacks its healthy cells, tissues, and organs. These conditions can cause chronic inflammation and damage, leading to long-term health problems.

It is worth noting that while some risk factors for chronic diseases are outside of our control (such as genetics), many others are modifiable through lifestyle changes, such as improving our diet, increasing physical activity, and quitting smoking.

D. The Impact of Chronic Diseases on Health

The impacts of chronic diseases on health can be significant and far-reaching, in terms of both physical health and overall quality of life. Here are some examples of the impacts of chronic diseases:

Physical limitations: Chronic diseases can limit a person's ability to perform everyday activities, such as walking, climbing stairs, or even getting dressed. They may also experience pain, stiffness, or weakness in various parts of the body.

Mental health issues: Chronic diseases can also have an impact on mental health, leading to depression, anxiety, and other psychological issues. This is often due to the limitations and challenges that come with managing a chronic disease.

Reduced life expectancy: Chronic diseases increase the risk of premature death, particularly if they are not properly managed or treated.

Financial burden: The cost of managing a chronic disease can be significant, including expenses for medications, doctor visits, and hospitalizations. This can cause financial strain for individuals and their families.

Social isolation: Chronic diseases can also impact a person's social life, as they may be unable to participate in certain activities or may feel stigmatized by their condition.

Increased risk of other health problems: Chronic diseases can give rise to the development of other health problems, such as infections, kidney disease, or eye problems. For example, people with diabetes are at increased risk of eye problems such as diabetic retinopathy, which can lead to vision loss.

Impact on family and caregivers: Chronic diseases can also affect the lives of family members and caregivers. These individuals may need to provide care, transportation, or emotional support for the person with the chronic disease, which can be draining both physically and emotionally.

Reduced productivity: Chronic diseases can also affect a person's ability to work or perform daily tasks, which can lead to reduced productivity and lost income.

Lower quality of life: Overall, chronic diseases can significantly reduce a person's quality of life, affecting their ability to engage in activities they enjoy, time spent with loved ones, and experience of a sense of purpose.

Increased healthcare utilization: Chronic diseases can also lead to increased use of healthcare services, including emergency room visits, hospitalizations, and specialist appointments. This can be a significant burden on the healthcare system and can contribute to rising healthcare costs.

In summary, chronic diseases can have a range of negative impacts on a person's physical, mental, and social well-being, as well as the well-being of their family and caregivers. Effective management and treatment of chronic diseases are essential to improve outcomes and quality of life for people living with these conditions.

E. Understanding the Conventional Approach to Treating Chronic Diseases

The first step in treating a chronic disease is typically to identify and diagnose the condition. This may involve a physical examination, blood tests, imaging studies, or other diagnostic tests. Once a diagnosis is made, a healthcare provider will develop a treatment plan based on the specific condition and the individual's health status and needs.

Medications are often a key component of treatment for chronic diseases. Different types of medications are available to manage symptoms, prevent complications, or slow the progression of the disease. For example, the use of medication to lower blood pressure in individuals with high blood pressure. In contrast, individuals with diabetes may be prescribed insulin or oral medications to help regulate their blood sugar levels.

Lifestyle changes are also an essential part of managing chronic diseases. Changes to diet, exercise, sleep, stress management, and other aspects of daily life are some of the lifestyle changes used in managing chronic diseases. For example, individuals with heart disease may be advised to maintain a low-fat diet, quit smoking, and engage in regular exercise to help manage their condition.

Ongoing monitoring is another critical component of treating chronic diseases. This may involve regular check-ups with a healthcare provider, blood tests or other diagnostic tests, or tracking symptoms and progress at home. Monitoring helps to ensure that the treatment plan is working effectively and can identify any potential complications or changes in the condition that require adjustment to the treatment plan.

In some cases, surgery or other more invasive treatments may be necessary to manage a chronic disease. For example, individuals with severe arthritis may require joint replacement surgery to improve their mobility and reduce pain.

Additional measures may include the following:

- **Patient Education:** In addition to medications, lifestyle changes, and monitoring, patient education is a critical component of treating chronic diseases. Healthcare providers will often educate patients on their condition, its causes, and its management strategies. Patients are typically encouraged to ask questions, seek support from their healthcare providers, and stay engaged in their treatment plan.

- **Multi-Disciplinary Approach:** Chronic diseases often require care from a team of healthcare providers, including primary care physicians, specialists, nurses, and other healthcare professionals. This team approach allows for more comprehensive care, with each provider bringing their expertise to the management of the condition.

- **Individualized Treatment Plans:** Every person is unique and will require a treatment plan that is tailored to their specific needs. Healthcare providers will consider factors such as age, gender, family history, lifestyle, and medical history when developing a treatment plan. This individualized approach ensures that patients receive the care that is best suited for them.

- **Continuous Improvement:** The conventional approach to treating chronic diseases is not static but rather an ongoing process of evaluating and adjusting treatment plans as necessary. Providers will monitor a patient's response to treatment, assess the effectiveness of medications and lifestyle changes, and make adjustments to ensure optimal management of the condition.

- **Complementary Therapies:** Along with conventional

approaches to treatment, complementary therapies, such as acupuncture, meditation, and yoga, can be used to manage chronic diseases. These therapies can help reduce stress, improve sleep quality, and promote overall wellness.

In conclusion, the conventional approach to treating chronic diseases is a comprehensive and ongoing process that aims to manage symptoms, prevent complications, and slow the progression of the disease. With a combination of medications, lifestyle changes, and ongoing monitoring, healthcare providers can help patients live longer, healthier lives with chronic diseases.

III: THE ROLE OF LIFESTYLE IN REVERSING CHRONIC DISEASES

A. Diet and Nutrition

Diet and nutrition play essential roles in preventing and treating chronic diseases. Chronic diseases are long-lasting health conditions that typically worsen over time, such as diabetes, heart disease, and cancer. A healthy diet, coupled with physical activity and other healthy lifestyle habits, can help prevent and manage chronic diseases.

Use of diet and nutrition in the treatment of chronic diseases:

1. **Type 2 diabetes:** Type 2 diabetes is a chronic disease that affects how the body processes glucose (sugar). A diet high in fiber, low in processed foods and added sugars and rich in whole grains, fruits, and vegetables can help regulate blood sugar levels and prevent complications. In some cases, medications may also be necessary to control blood sugar.

2. **Heart disease:** Heart disease is a leading cause of death worldwide. A heart-healthy diet should include plenty of fruits, vegetables, whole grains, lean proteins, and healthy fats. Limiting salt, sugar, saturated and trans fats is also necessary. Physical activity, smoking cessation, and managing stress can also help prevent and manage heart disease.

3. **Cancer:** While there is no specific 'cancer diet', a healthy, balanced diet that is rich in fruits, vegetables, whole grains, and lean proteins can help reduce the risk of certain types of cancer. Some studies suggest that certain foods, such as cruciferous vegetables (like broccoli and cauliflower) and berries, may have cancer-fighting properties.

4. **Chronic kidney disease:** A diet that is low in sodium, protein, and phosphorus can help slow the progression of chronic kidney disease. Eating plenty of fruits and vegetables can also provide necessary nutrients while limiting potassium and phosphorus.

5. **Inflammatory Bowel Disease (IBD):** IBD is a chronic condition that causes inflammation in the digestive tract. While there is no one-size-fits-all diet for IBD, some people find that certain foods can trigger flare-ups. Keeping a food diary and working with a registered dietitian can help identify trigger foods and develop a personalized diet plan.

6. **Osteoporosis:** Osteoporosis is a condition in which bones become brittle and weak, increasing the risk of fractures. Adequate calcium and vitamin D intake is crucial for bone health, and a diet rich in these can help prevent osteoporosis. Good dietary sources of calcium include dairy products, leafy green vegetables, and fortified foods. Sunlight, fortified foods, and supplements are good sources of vitamin D.

7. **Arthritis:** Arthritis is a common chronic condition that causes joint pain and inflammation. A healthy diet rich in fruits, vegetables, whole grains, and lean proteins can help reduce inflammation and improve joint health. Some

studies have also suggested that omega-3 fatty acids in fatty fish like salmon may help reduce joint pain.

8. **Multiple Sclerosis (MS):** MS is a chronic condition that affects the nervous system. While there is no specific diet for MS, some researchers suggest that a diet low in saturated fat and high in fruits, vegetables, and whole grains may help reduce inflammation and improve overall health.

9. **Chronic Obstructive Pulmonary Disease (COPD):** COPD is a chronic lung condition that can make breathing difficult. A healthy diet rich in fruits, vegetables, and whole grains can provide necessary nutrients and improve lung function. It is important to maintain a healthy weight for managing COPD; as excess weight can make breathing more difficult.

10. **Irritable Bowel Syndrome (IBS):** IBS is a chronic digestive disorder that can cause abdominal pain, bloating, and changes in bowel habits. Some people find that certain foods, such as high-fat or spicy foods, can trigger symptoms. Working with a registered dietitian to identify trigger foods and develop a personalized diet plan can help manage symptoms and improve overall health.

In addition to the afore-mentioned chronic diseases, diet, and nutrition can also be used to manage other conditions, such as high blood pressure, high cholesterol, and obesity. It is important to note that while diet and nutrition can play an essential role in the prevention and management of chronic diseases, they should not replace medications or other treatments prescribed by a healthcare provider. A healthy diet and lifestyle should be used in conjunction with other medical treatments to achieve the best possible health outcomes.

B. Exercise and Physical activity

Regular exercise and physical activity are effective in reversing chronic diseases, which are long-term conditions that persist over time and are often characterized by progressive worsening of symptoms. These conditions include heart disease, diabetes, hypertension, obesity, and certain types of cancer, among others.

In the case of heart disease, exercise, and physical activity have been shown to improve heart function, reduce blood pressure and cholesterol levels, and improve overall cardiovascular health. Exercise can also help reduce the risk of developing heart disease in the first place.

Similarly, regular physical activity can help manage and even reverse type 2 diabetes. Exercise helps the body use insulin more efficiently. Chronic inflammation is like a constant, low-level alarm in your body. It's when your body's defense system stays active for a long time, even when there's no immediate threat. This can lead to health problems over time. This lowers blood sugar levels and reduces the risk of developing diabetes-related complications such as nerve damage and kidney disease.

In addition to heart disease and diabetes, exercise and physical activity can also help reverse other chronic conditions. For example, regular exercise can help lower blood pressure in people with hypertension. It can also help manage symptoms of depression and anxiety. Exercise can also be an effective tool for managing and reversing obesity, which is a risk factor for many chronic diseases.

The key to using exercise and physical activity to reverse chronic diseases is consistency. It is crucial to engage in regular, moderate-intensity physical activity on most days of the week, and to increase the duration and intensity of exercise over time gradually. It is also essential to develop an exercise plan that is safe and appropriate for your individual needs, taking into account any health conditions or limitations.

In addition to exercise, other lifestyle factors such as diet and stress management can also play a role in reversing chronic diseases. A healthy, balanced diet that is rich in fruits, vegetables, whole grains, and lean protein can help support overall health and well-being. Stress management techniques such as meditation, yoga, and deep breathing exercises can also help manage chronic diseases and improve overall health.

In summary, regular exercise and physical activity can be a powerful tool in reversing chronic diseases, including heart disease, diabetes, hypertension, obesity, and more. By working with a healthcare provider to develop a safe and appropriate exercise plan and by making healthy lifestyle choices such as eating a balanced diet and managing stress, it is possible to improve overall health, well-being and potentially even reverse chronic diseases.

In addition to the health benefits discussed above, exercise and physical activity can also improve overall quality of life, including increased energy, better sleep, and reduced stress levels. These benefits can have a positive impact on mental health, emotional well-being, and social interactions, which further support overall health and well-being.

For people with chronic diseases, regular exercise and physical activity can help reduce symptoms and improve functional ability. For example, people with arthritis can benefit from regular exercises, which reduce pain, improve function and mobility in the joints. Exercise also helps people with chronic obstructive pulmonary disease (COPD) breathe easier and improve their ability to perform daily activities.

It is important to note that exercise and physical activity are not a one-size-fits-all solution, and what works for one person may not work for another. The type and intensity of exercise should be tailored to the individual's specific needs and abilities, and any limitations or health concerns should be taken into account.

It is also important to start slowly and gradually increase the duration and intensity of exercise over time. This can help prevent injury and avoid burnout. It is also a good idea to mix up the type of exercise to keep things interesting and prevent boredom.

Finally, physical activity does not necessarily have to involve structured exercise such as going to the gym or taking a fitness class. Activities such as gardening, walking, dancing, and playing with children or pets can all be great ways to incorporate physical activity into daily life.

Overall, exercise and physical activity are powerful tools for improving health and well-being and can play an essential role in reversing chronic diseases. By working with a healthcare provider to develop a safe and appropriate exercise plan and by making healthy lifestyle choices, it is possible to live a healthier, happier, and more active life.

C. Stress Management

Stress is a common factor that affects many aspects of a person's life, including physical health. High levels of stress often or exacerbate chronic diseases such as diabetes, heart disease, and obesity. In order to reverse chronic diseases, it is vital to manage stress effectively. Below are some tips for stress management that can help in reversing chronic diseases:

- **Identify and manage the causes of stress:** The first step in stress management is to identify the cause of stress. Keeping a stress diary helps you to identify patterns and triggers of stress. Once you have identified the causes of stress, you can then take steps to manage or eliminate them.
- **Practice relaxation techniques:** Relaxation techniques such as deep breathing, yoga, and meditation can help to reduce stress and promote relaxation. Incorporate these into your daily routines to help manage stress.
- **Get regular exercise:** Exercise is a powerful stress reliever that also has numerous health benefits. Regular exercise

can help to reduce stress, improve mood, and promote overall health. It is necessary to find an exercise routine that is enjoyable and sustainable.

- **Get enough sleep:** Chronic stress can disrupt sleep patterns and in turn, exacerbate chronic diseases. Getting enough sleep is crucial for stress management and overall health. Aim for 7-9 hours of sleep per night and establish a regular sleep schedule.
- **Eat a healthy diet:** A healthy diet can help to reduce stress and promote overall health. Eating a balanced diet that is rich in fruits, vegetables, whole grains, and lean protein provides the nutrients needed for stress management and disease reversal.
- **Seek support:** Chronic diseases can be overwhelming, and it is important to seek support from family, friends, or a professional therapist. Talking about stress and the challenges of managing chronic diseases helps to reduce stress and provide a sense of emotional support.
- **Set realistic goals:** Setting goals and breaking them down into smaller, achievable steps can help to reduce stress and prevent burnout. It is essential to set goals that are realistic and achievable, rather than overwhelming.
- **Practice self-care:** Taking time for self-care activities, such as reading a book, taking a bath, or going for a walk, can help to reduce stress and promote relaxation. Self-care activities can also improve mood and overall well-being.
- **Practice mindfulness:** Mindfulness is the practice of being present and fully engaged in the current moment. Mindfulness techniques, such as deep breathing, meditation, or simply focusing on the present moment, can help to reduce stress and promote relaxation.
- **Practice time management:** Poor time management can lead to increased stress and anxiety. It is important to prioritize tasks and manage time effectively to reduce stress and increase productivity.
- **Practice gratitude:** Practicing gratitude, or focusing on

the positive aspects of life, can help to reduce stress and promote emotional well-being. Taking time each day to focus on the things you are grateful for can help to shift your perspective and reduce stress.

- **Reduce caffeine and alcohol consumption:** Caffeine and alcohol worsen stress and anxiety, so it is essential to consume these substances in moderation or possibly eliminate them outrightly.

By practicing these stress management techniques, you can promote disease reversal and overall well-being. Remember that stress management is a lifelong journey, and it is important to continue to make small changes and adjustments to find what works best for you. There is a need for patience and consistency.

D. Sleep and Rest

Getting enough sleep and rest can be a crucial factor in reversing chronic diseases. Long-term or recurring health conditions typically characterize chronic diseases, and they can include a wide range of conditions such as heart disease, diabetes, cancer, and autoimmune disorders.

Research has shown that sleep and rest play a vital role in maintaining our overall health. Chronic sleep deprivation and poor sleep quality can contribute to the development and progression of chronic diseases. Lack of sleep has been linked to an increased risk of heart disease, stroke, diabetes, obesity, and certain cancers.

Getting adequate rest and sleep can help to improve the body's natural healing processes, reduce inflammation, and boost the immune system. This is important because chronic diseases often involve chronic inflammation, which can lead to tissue damage and further exacerbate the disease.

One of the ways that sleep helps to reverse chronic diseases is by supporting the body's natural healing processes. During sleep, the body releases growth hormones that promote tissue repair and regeneration. Chronic diseases often involve damage to tissues and organs; so getting enough sleep helps the body repair and heal this damage.

Sleep also plays a critical role in regulating the immune system, which is important for people with chronic diseases. Research has shown that sleep deprivation can suppress the immune system, making it more difficult for the body to fight off infections and other threats. On the other hand, getting enough sleep strengthens the immune system and improves its ability to respond to infections and other challenges.

Another way that sleep helps reverse chronic diseases is by reducing inflammation. Chronic inflammation is a common factor in many chronic diseases, and it contributes to tissue damage and other adverse effects. Research has shown that getting enough sleep can reduce inflammation in the body, which then helps to improve overall health and well-being.

Rest is also advisable for people with chronic diseases. Rest takes many forms, including physical rest, mental rest, and emotional rest. Physical rest involves taking time to relax and recover from physical activity. In contrast, mental and emotional rest involve reducing stress, practicing mindfulness, and engaging in activities that promote relaxation and calm.

Chronic diseases are stressful and emotionally tasking, so taking time for rest is particularly important for people dealing with these conditions. Research has shown that stress and emotional turmoil have adverse effects on the immune system and contribute to chronic inflammation. Taking steps to reduce stress and promote relaxation an important part of reversing chronic diseases.

In summary, getting enough sleep and rest is a critical factor in reversing chronic diseases. By supporting the body's natural healing processes, regulating the immune system, reducing inflammation, and promoting relaxation, sleep, and rest help people with chronic diseases to improve their overall health and well-being.

In dealing with chronic diseases, it is important to work closely with your healthcare provider to develop a comprehensive treatment plan that addresses all aspects of your health, including sleep, rest, diet, and exercise. By taking a holistic approach, you can reverse the progression of your chronic disease and improve your overall quality of life.

E. Environmental Factors

Chronic diseases, such as heart disease, diabetes, and cancer, are often caused by a complex interplay of genetic, lifestyle, and environmental factors. While genetics play a role in the development of chronic diseases, environmental factors also have a significant impact, and modifying these factors can help to reverse or prevent the onset of chronic diseases.

Some environmental factors that contribute to chronic diseases and ways to reverse their impact are discussed below:

Air pollution

Exposure to air pollution has been linked to a variety of chronic diseases, including heart disease, stroke, and lung cancer. Reducing exposure to air pollution by avoiding heavily trafficked areas or using air purifiers can help reverse the impact of air pollution on health.

Diet

- **Resource Consumption:** The type of diet we follow can

have a significant impact on the environment. Diets high in meat and processed foods often require more resources like land, water, and energy compared to plant-based diets.

- **Greenhouse Gas Emissions**: Meat production, in particular, contributes to substantial greenhouse gas emissions. Adopting a more plant-based diet can reduce these emissions.
- **Sustainable Agriculture**: Supporting sustainable farming practices, such as organic farming and reducing food waste, can lessen the environmental impact of our diet.

Physical Activity

- **Transportation**: How we choose to move from one place to another affects the environment. Using public transportation, carpooling, walking, or cycling can reduce carbon emissions compared to using personal vehicles.
- **Outdoor Recreation**: Enjoying physical activities in natural settings requires preserving and protecting these areas to minimize habitat destruction and maintain biodiversity.

Stress

- **Consumerism**: Stress can lead to overconsumption and a "throwaway culture." This can result in more production, resource use, and waste, impacting the environment. Encouraging a more mindful and less consumer-driven lifestyle can reduce this effect.

Sleep

- **Energy Use**: Sleep habits can indirectly affect the environment through energy consumption. Leaving lights and electronic devices on unnecessarily can lead to increased energy use. Implementing energy-saving practices at home can mitigate this impact.
- **Circadian Rhythms**: Disrupted sleep patterns due to excessive artificial light at night can affect wildlife, particularly nocturnal animals. Reducing light pollution

can help protect ecosystems.

Exposure to chemicals

Exposure to chemicals found in food, water, household products, and personal care products are linked to a variety of chronic diseases. Reducing exposure to these chemicals by choosing organic foods using non-toxic household and personal care products can help reverse the impact of chemical exposure on health.

Social support

Social isolation and lack of support are responsible for chronic diseases such as depression, anxiety, and heart disease. Building a solid support network, such as friends, family, or support groups, can help reverse the impact of social isolation on health.

Environmental toxins

Exposure to environmental toxins, such as pesticides and heavy metals, has been linked to chronic diseases such as cancer and neurological disorders. Reducing exposure to these toxins by avoiding contaminated foods, using water filters, and choosing non-toxic household and personal care products can help reverse the impact of environmental toxins on health.

Avoiding unnecessary exposure to radiation, mainly from our communication masts and high tension electricity lines located around residential areas, would go a long way too.

Smoking and secondhand smoke

Smoking and exposure to secondhand smoke can lead to chronic diseases such as lung cancer, heart disease, and stroke. Quitting smoking and avoiding exposure to secondhand smoke can help reverse the impact of smoking on health.

Occupational hazards

Exposure to occupational hazards, such as chemicals, dust, and radiation, is responsible for a number of chronic diseases such as lung disease and cancer. Reducing exposure to these hazards through workplace safety measures can reverse the impact of occupational hazards on health.

Climate change

Climate change plays an important role in the onset of chronic diseases such as asthma, heat-related illnesses, and infectious diseases. The reduction of carbon emissions and promotion of sustainable practices can reverse the impact of climate change on health.

It is important to note that environmental factors are capable of interacting with genetic and lifestyle factors to impact chronic disease risk and reversal. Therefore, a holistic approach that considers all of these factors is necessary for effective chronic disease prevention and management.

In summary, our choices as far as these environment factors are concerned can collectively have a significant impact on health. Adopting sustainable practices, reducing resource consumption, and being mindful of our lifestyle choices can contribute to a healthier and more environmentally friendly world.

In conclusion, modification of environmental factors is an important step in reversing their impact on chronic diseases. It is important to note that these changes may take time and require sustained effort to achieve long-lasting results.

F. Importance of Lifestyle Changes in Reversing Chronic Diseases.

Chronic diseases, such as type 2 diabetes, cardiovascular disease, and obesity, are becoming increasingly prevalent worldwide. Lifestyle factors such as poor diet, physical inactivity, and tobacco and alcohol use are often responsible for these conditions. While medical interventions such as medication and surgery can be effective in managing symptoms, lifestyle changes are crucial for reversing these chronic diseases and improving overall health.

Making lifestyle changes such as adopting a healthy diet, increasing physical activity, reducing stress, and quitting smoking and excessive alcohol consumption can have significant positive effects on chronic diseases. These changes cause reduction in symptoms and improve overall health outcomes, including weight loss, improved blood sugar control, lowered blood pressure, and reduced cholesterol levels. In some cases, these changes can even lead to remission or complete reversal of the disease.

For instance, in the case of type 2 diabetes, adopting a healthy diet and increasing physical activity improves insulin sensitivity, which in turn leads to improved blood sugar control. Similarly, in the case of cardiovascular disease, lifestyle changes such as adopting a healthy diet and quitting smoking reduces the risk of heart attack and stroke.

It is important to note that making lifestyle changes is challenging, and takes time and effort to see significant improvements in health outcomes. However, with the support of healthcare professionals, family and friends, it is possible to make sustainable changes that can lead to long-term health benefits.

Reduction/elimination of medication

While medication helps in managing symptoms of chronic diseases, making lifestyle changes can reduce the need for or eliminate the need for it. For example, in some cases, making healthy lifestyle changes helps individuals with high blood pressure reduce dependence or even stop taking medication.

Preventing chronic diseases from developing

Making healthy lifestyle changes can help prevent chronic diseases from developing in the first place. Eating a healthy diet, engaging in regular physical activity, and quitting smoking, for example, reduces the risk of developing type 2 diabetes, cardiovascular disease, and certain types of cancer.

Effects of lifestyle changes on mental health

Making lifestyle changes can have positive effects on mental health as well. For example, engaging in regular physical activity can reduce symptoms of depression and anxiety, while practicing stress-reducing techniques such as meditation and deep breathing can help improve overall mood and reduce stress.

Improvement in quality of life

Reversing chronic diseases through lifestyle changes can significantly improve quality of life. For example, individuals who adopt a healthy lifestyle may have more energy, improved sleep, and reduced pain and discomfort.

Sustainability

Making lifestyle changes can be a long-term and sustainable way to manage chronic diseases. By adopting a healthy lifestyle, individuals can make lasting changes that lead to improved health outcomes and reduce the risk of chronic diseases in the future.

In summary, making lifestyle changes is essential for reversing chronic diseases and improving overall health outcomes. These changes help reduce the need for medication, prevent chronic diseases from developing, improve mental health, quality of life, and can be sustainable for the long term.

In conclusion, lifestyle changes are crucial for reversing chronic diseases and improving overall health outcomes. By adopting a healthy diet, increasing physical activity, reducing stress, and quitting smoking and excessive alcohol consumption, individuals can experience significant improvements in their health and reduce the risk of chronic diseases.

IV: NATURAL AND ALTERNATIVE THERAPIES FOR REVERSING CHRONIC DISEASES

A. Herbs and Supplements

Herbs and supplements can help manage and potentially reverse chronic diseases. Still, it is important to note that they should not be a replacement for medical treatment or advice from a healthcare professional.

Some herbs and supplements studied for their potentials in managing and reversing chronic diseases:

Curcumin

Curcumin is a compound found in the spice turmeric and has been studied for its potential anti-inflammatory and antioxidant effects. Research has shown that curcumin plays a role in reducing inflammation in conditions such as arthritis and also has the potential to manage chronic conditions such as diabetes, heart disease, and cancer.

Omega-3 fatty acids

Omega-3 fatty acids, found in fish oil supplements and certain foods like fatty fish, have been shown to have anti-inflammatory properties and may have potential in managing conditions such as rheumatoid arthritis, inflammatory bowel disease, and heart disease.

Ginseng

Ginseng has been used in traditional medicine for its potential immune-boosting and anti-inflammatory effects. Some studies have shown that ginseng may have the potential to manage conditions such as diabetes, heart disease, and cancer.

Probiotics

Probiotics are live bacteria and yeasts that are beneficial for gut health. They have been studied for their potential to improve conditions such as irritable bowel syndrome, inflammatory bowel disease, and some allergies.

Green Tea

Green tea contains compounds called catechins, which have been studied for their potential anti-inflammatory and antioxidant effects. Some studies have shown that green tea may have the potential to manage conditions such as heart disease and cancer.

Garlic

Garlic has been used for centuries for its potential health benefits, including its anti-inflammatory, antioxidant, and immune-boosting properties. Research has shown that garlic may help manage conditions such as high blood pressure, high cholesterol, and certain types of cancer.

Milk thistle

Milk thistle is a herb that has been traditionally used to support liver function. Some research has shown that milk thistle may have the potential to manage liver conditions such as hepatitis and cirrhosis.

Coenzyme Q10 (CoQ10)

CoQ10 is a compound found in every cell of the body and is involved in producing energy. Some research has shown that CoQ10 may have the potential to manage conditions such as heart disease, Parkinson's disease, and migraines.

Magnesium

Magnesium is an essential mineral that is involved in over 300 biochemical reactions in the body. It is crucial for maintaining healthy bones, regulating blood sugar levels, and supporting a healthy nervous system. Research shows that magnesium may help manage conditions such as high blood pressure, type 2 diabetes, and migraine headaches.

Vitamin D

Vitamin D is a fat-soluble vitamin that is important for bone health and immune function. Research has shown that vitamin D is important in the management of conditions such as osteoporosis, multiple sclerosis, and some types of cancer.

It is important to note that while some herbs and supplements may have potential benefits in managing chronic diseases, they can also interact with medications and may have potential side effects. It is important to talk to a healthcare professional before starting any new supplement or herb.

True prevention medicine involves encouraging and supporting patients to take a threefold approach:

1. Eat healthy

2. Practice a consistent exercise program

3. Embrace consuming high-quality nutritional supplements.

Therefore, empowering people to avoid getting any major disease in the first place is true prevention.

B. Acupuncture and Massage

Acupuncture and massage therapy are alternative medical practices that have been used for centuries to treat a variety of health conditions, including chronic diseases. While some studies suggest that acupuncture and massage therapy may have some benefits in managing symptoms associated with certain chronic diseases, the evidence supporting their ability to reverse chronic diseases is limited.

Chronic diseases are typically caused by a combination of genetic, environmental, and lifestyle factors; reversing them requires addressing the underlying causes. Acupuncture and massage therapy may help alleviate symptoms associated with chronic diseases, such as pain, anxiety, and depression. However, they are unlikely to reverse the course of the disease itself.

Incorporating acupuncture and massage therapy into an overall treatment plan for chronic diseases may be beneficial for some patients. These therapies help manage symptoms, reduce stress, and improve overall well-being, which then contribute to a better overall health and quality of life.

Acupuncture is a form of Traditional Chinese Medicine that involves inserting thin needles into specific points on the body. The theory behind acupuncture is that it helps to balance the body's energy, or 'Qi', and stimulate the body's natural healing processes. It has been used to treat a variety of conditions, including chronic pain, anxiety, and depression.

Several studies have suggested that acupuncture may be beneficial for managing symptoms associated with chronic diseases. A 2018 systematic review and meta-analysis of randomized controlled trials found that acupuncture was effective in reducing pain in patients with chronic lower back pain, osteoarthritis, and chronic headaches. Another systematic review of randomized controlled trials showed that acupuncture was effective in reducing symptoms of anxiety and depression in patients with chronic illnesses.

Massage therapy is another alternative medical practice that involves manipulating the body's soft tissues, such as muscles and connective tissue. It has been used to treat a variety of conditions, including chronic pain, anxiety, and depression.

Several studies suggest that massage therapy may be beneficial for managing symptoms associated with chronic diseases. A 2015 systematic review of randomized controlled trials found that massage therapy was effective in reducing pain and improving quality of life in patients with chronic low back pain. Another systematic review of randomized controlled trials found that the therapy was effective in reducing symptoms of anxiety and depression in patients with chronic illnesses.

In summary, while there is evidence to suggest that acupuncture and massage therapy are beneficial for managing symptoms associated with chronic diseases, the evidence supporting their ability to reverse chronic diseases is limited. These therapies should be used in conjunction with other medical treatments, such as medication and lifestyle changes. They are not a substitute for medical care. It is crucial to work with a qualified healthcare professional to determine the most appropriate treatment plan for your specific condition.

C. Meditation and Mindfulness

Studies show that meditation and mindfulness practices have a positive impact on various chronic diseases. These practices help reduce stress and anxiety, improve mood, enhance the immune system, and reduce inflammation in the body.

Examples of chronic diseases affected positively by meditation and mindfulness:

Cardiovascular disease

Meditation and mindfulness practices have been shown to reduce blood pressure, lower cholesterol levels, and decrease the risk of heart disease. Stress is a significant contributor to cardiovascular disease. Meditation and mindfulness practices help to reduce stress, which in turn lowers blood pressure and improves heart health. One study found that people who practiced Transcendental Meditation had a 48% reduction in their risk of heart attack, stroke, and death compared to a control group.

Diabetes

Mindfulness-based interventions have been found to improve blood sugar levels, reduce insulin resistance, and improve overall health in people with diabetes. Stress is also a factor in diabetes management. When the body is under stress, it releases cortisol, which causes blood sugar levels to rise. Mindfulness practices reduce stress and lowers cortisol levels, leading to better blood sugar control.

Chronic pain

Mindfulness-based stress reduction (MBSR) has been shown to improve pain symptoms in people with chronic pain conditions such as fibromyalgia, arthritis, and back pain. Chronic pain can be taxing both physically and mentally. Mindfulness-based interventions can help people with chronic pain to manage their pain better, reduce stress and anxiety, and improve overall well-being. One study found that participants who practiced MBSR reported a 40% reduction in pain intensity and a 57% reduction in disability.

Depression and anxiety

Mindfulness-based cognitive therapy (MBCT) is effective in reducing symptoms of depression and anxiety. Depression and anxiety have negative impact on physical health as well. Mindfulness-based therapies contribute to improvement in mood and reduction in the symptoms of depression and anxiety. An improved overall well-being is the final outcome. One study found that MBCT was just as effective as antidepressant medication in preventing relapse in people with recurrent depression.

Cancer

Meditation and mindfulness practices have been found to improve quality of life and reduce symptoms in cancer patients. Cancer treatment, as well, can be taxing physically and emotionally. Meditation and mindfulness practices have been found to improve quality of life and reduce symptoms such as anxiety, depression, and fatigue in cancer patients. One study found that a mindfulness-based intervention reduced symptoms of anxiety and depression in breast cancer patients undergoing chemotherapy.

In general, meditation and mindfulness practices help to improve overall well-being and quality of life, which can be particularly important for people with chronic diseases. They also help to promote relaxation, reduce stress and anxiety, and improve immune function, all of which support the body's natural healing processes.

D. Home remedies and folk medicine

Home remedies and folk medicine have been used for centuries to treat various ailments, including chronic diseases. While these practices can provide some relief, it's important to note that they are no substitutes for professional medical advice and treatment. Here are some examples of home remedies and folk medicine for specific chronic conditions:

- **Arthritis**: Some people believe in the efficacy of consuming ginger or turmeric to alleviate joint pain and inflammation. These spices contain compounds with anti-inflammatory properties.

- **Asthma**: Honey and warm water are often used to soothe the throat and potentially reduce coughing in people with asthma. Honey may have mild anti-inflammatory effects.
- **Diabetes**: Bitter melon is a popular folk remedy for diabetes management. Some studies suggest it may help lower blood sugar levels. However, it's not a replacement for prescribed medications and dietary control.
- **Hypertension**: Garlic is believed to have blood pressure-lowering properties. Some individuals incorporate garlic into their diets or consume garlic supplements.
- **Digestive Issues**: Ginger and peppermint are used to relieve various digestive problems like nausea, indigestion, and irritable bowel syndrome. They can have calming effects on the stomach.
- **Headaches**: Aromatherapy with essential oils like lavender or peppermint may be used to alleviate tension headaches. Peppermint oil can be applied topically for a cooling sensation.
- **Skin Conditions**: Aloe vera is often applied typically to soothe skin conditions like psoriasis and eczema due to its potential anti-inflammatory properties.

It's important to emphasize that these remedies should be used cautiously, and their effects can vary from person to person. Always consult with a healthcare professional to create a comprehensive and evidence-based treatment plan for chronic diseases. Folk remedies can complement medical treatments, but they should not replace them. Additionally, some folk remedies may have side effects or interact with prescribed medications, so it's essential to consult a healthcare provider before trying them.

Chronic diseases are complex conditions that often require medical intervention and management by qualified healthcare professionals. However, some home remedies and folk medicine practices have been studied and found to have potential health benefits in managing or preventing chronic diseases. For example, incorporating certain herbs and spices into your diet may help reduce inflammation and improve blood sugar control in people with diabetes. Some common examples include cinnamon, turmeric, and ginger.

Some of the practices include:

Acupuncture

Acupuncture is an ancient Chinese healing technique that involves inserting thin needles into specific points on the body. Studies have shown that acupuncture may help manage chronic pain, reduce stress, and improve sleep. However, more research is needed to determine its effectiveness for other chronic diseases.

Mind-body practices

Mind-body practices, such as meditation, yoga, and tai chi, have been shown to reduce stress and improve overall well-being. These practices may also help manage chronic conditions, such as heart disease, diabetes, and chronic pain.

Herbal supplements

Some herbal supplements, such as ginseng, garlic, and St. John's wort, have been shown to have potential health benefits for certain chronic conditions. However, it is important to speak with a healthcare provider before taking any supplements, as some can interact with medications or cause side effects.

Dietary modifications

Making dietary modifications, such as reducing sugar and processed foods and increasing intake of fruits and vegetables can help manage chronic conditions such as diabetes, heart disease, and high blood pressure. It is essential to work with a healthcare provider or a registered dietitian to develop an individualized dietary plan.

Traditional Chinese Medicine

Traditional Chinese Medicine (TCM) includes practices such as herbal medicine, acupuncture, massage, and dietary therapy. TCM has been used for thousands of years to manage a variety of chronic conditions. While some TCM practices may have potential health benefits, it is important to speak with a qualified TCM practitioner and a healthcare provider before trying any TCM treatments.

It is important to note that while some home remedies and folk medicine practices may have potential health benefits, they should not be a replacement for evidence-based medical treatments. A balanced approach that incorporates both traditional medical treatments and healthy lifestyle modifications may be the most effective way to manage chronic diseases.

E. Scientific basis for Natural and alternative therapies

Natural and alternative therapies encompass a wide range of treatments and interventions that are typically outside the scope of conventional medicine. The scientific basis for these therapies varies widely, and it's essential to evaluate each one individually. Here, I'll discuss the scientific basis for some commonly used natural and alternative therapies, but keep in mind that the efficacy of these therapies can vary, and not all have strong scientific support.

Acupuncture

Numerous studies have shown that acupuncture can be effective in treating a variety of conditions, such as chronic pain, headaches, and nausea. It involves the insertion of thin needles into specific points on the body to alleviate various conditions.

While the exact mechanisms are not fully understood, some studies suggest that acupuncture can trigger the release of endorphins and modulate the nervous system, providing pain relief and other benefits.

Herbal medicine

Herbal medicine involves the use of plants or plant extracts to treat various conditions. While some herbal remedies are effective in clinical trials, others are yet to be well-studied and may have adverse effects.

Many pharmaceutical drugs are derived from plants, which suggests that there is scientific merit in exploring the potential benefits of herbal remedies.

Some herbal medicines, like St. John's Wort for depression or Echinacea for immune support, have been studied, and there is evidence of their effectiveness.

Meditation

Meditation involves the practice of focusing your attention on a specific object, thought, or activity to achieve a state of calmness and relaxation. Studies have shown that meditation can help reduce stress, anxiety, and depression.

Chiropractic

Chiropractic is a complementary and alternative medicine practice that involves the manipulation of the spine and other joints to alleviate pain and improve function. It focuses on the musculoskeletal system, primarily spinal adjustments to alleviate pain and improve health. While some studies have shown that chiropractic can be effective in treating certain types of pain, other studies have found little or no benefit.

Scientific evidence for chiropractic care is mixed, with some studies suggesting benefits for certain conditions like lower back pain. In contrast, others question its effectiveness for various health issues.

Aromatherapy

Aromatherapy involves the use of essential oils to promote relaxation, improve mood, and alleviate pain. While some studies have shown that certain essential oils can be effective for these purposes, more research is needed to understand their potential benefits fully.

Yoga

Yoga involves the practice of physical postures, breathing exercises, and meditation to improve physical and mental health. Numerous studies have shown that yoga can help reduce stress, anxiety, and depression, as well as improve flexibility, strength, and balance.

Mindfulness-based interventions:

Mindfulness-based interventions are techniques that focus on being present in the moment and non-judgmentally accepting one's thoughts, feelings, and sensations. These techniques are effective in reducing stress, anxiety, and depression, as well as improving overall well-being.

Practices like meditation and mindfulness have been extensively studied, and there's strong scientific evidence supporting their efficacy in reducing anxiety, stress and improving overall mental well-being.

Studies have shown changes in brain structure and function associated with regular meditation practice.

Homeopathy

Homeopathy is a controversial therapy based on the principle of "like cures like" and extreme dilution of substances.

It is a system of medicine that involves the use of highly diluted substances to stimulate the body's natural healing process. While some studies have found that homeopathy can be effective for certain conditions, other studies, including scientific consensus is essentially against homeopathy due to the lack of plausible mechanisms and consistent evidence of its effectiveness beyond a placebo effect.

Traditional Chinese Medicine (TCM)

Traditional Chinese medicine is a system of medicine that includes acupuncture, herbal medicine, and other practices. While some TCM practices have been found to be effective in clinical trials, others have yet to be well studied and may have adverse effects.

TCM includes practices like acupuncture, herbal medicine, and qi gong. Some components of TCM have scientific support, such as acupuncture, while others lack rigorous scientific validation.

Ayurveda

Ayurveda is an ancient Indian system of medicine that includes herbal remedies, dietary recommendations, and

lifestyle practices.

Some Ayurvedic herbs and practices have been researched, but the scientific basis varies depending on the specific intervention.

Naturopathy

Naturopathic medicine combines various natural therapies, emphasizing a holistic approach to health.

The scientific basis for naturopathy varies by the specific treatments. It may include both evidence-based practices and less substantiated interventions.

Naturopathic medicine is an alternative medical system that focuses on natural remedies and the body's ability to heal itself. While some naturopathic treatments, such as dietary changes and stress reduction techniques, are effective, other treatments, such as homeopathy, have been found to have little scientific basis.

Energy healing

Energy healing is a group of alternative therapies that involve the manipulation of energy fields to promote healing. While some forms of energy healing, such as Reiki, have been found to be effective in reducing pain and anxiety, the scientific basis for these therapies is still under debate.

It is important to note that while some natural and alternative therapies have a solid scientific basis, others may not be supported by rigorous scientific evidence. It is always a good idea to do your research and talk to a healthcare professional before trying any new therapy,especially if you have any medical conditions or are taking any medications.

F. How to determine the right natural and alternative therapies for your specific needs

Determining the right natural and alternative therapies for your specific needs can be a complex process, and it is important to approach it with care and attention to your individual health needs. Here are some steps you can take to help determine which therapies might be suitable for you:

Please consult with a healthcare professional: It is important to talk to your healthcare provider before starting any natural or alternative therapy to ensure it is safe for you and won't interfere with any existing medical conditions or medications.

Please do your research: Look up information about different natural and alternative therapies and their benefits, risks, and any possible side effects. Be wary of unverified or misleading information.

Consider your health goals: Think about what you hope to achieve by using natural or alternative therapies. For example, are you looking to manage chronic pain, reduce stress, or improve your sleep? Knowing your goals can help you select the right therapy.

Assess your preferences: Consider the delivery method of the therapy. Would you prefer a supplement, herbal remedy, massage, or acupuncture? Consider what you are most comfortable with.

Seek out a qualified practitioner: If you choose to work with a practitioner, make sure they have the proper credentials and experience to provide the therapy. Feel free to ask for references or reviews.

Keep track of your progress: Keep track of how the therapy is working for you, and be willing to make adjustments or try a different therapy if needed.

Understand the science behind the therapy: Look for evidence-based information about the therapy you're considering. While not all natural and alternative therapies have been extensively studied, many have research backing up their effectiveness.

Consider the potential risks and side effects: Just because a therapy is natural does not mean it is completely safe. Some natural therapies can interact with medications or may not be safe for people with certain medical conditions. Be sure to research potential side effects and risks associated with any therapy you are considering.

Take into account your overall lifestyle: Your overall lifestyle can affect your health and wellness. Therefore, consider how changes to your diet, exercise routine, and stress management practices can influence your health in addition to any natural or alternative therapies you are considering.

Be patient and consistent: Natural and alternative therapies often take time to work, so be patient and consistent with your chosen therapy. It is essential to follow the recommended dosage or treatment plan and give the therapy time to work before deciding if it is right for you.

Trust your instincts: Ultimately, the decision to try a natural or alternative therapy is up to you. If something does not feel right or you have concerns, listen to your instincts and consult with your healthcare provider.

Determining the suitable natural and alternative therapies for your specific needs requires a holistic approach that takes into account your unique health needs, lifestyle, and preferences. By doing your research, consulting with healthcare providers, and taking a thoughtful approach, you can identify the therapies that may be most effective for you.

V:WORKING WITH HEALTHCARE PROVIDERS

A. Importance of Collaboration with Healthcare Providers

Collaboration with healthcare providers is essential for improving patient outcomes and delivering high-quality health care. Healthcare providers, including doctors, pharmacists, nurses, and other medical professionals, bring different areas of expertise and experience to patient care. By working together, they can ensure that patients receive comprehensive care that addresses their unique needs and challenges.

Here are some key reasons why collaboration with healthcare providers is so important:

Comprehensive care

Healthcare providers are able to provide a more comprehensive approach to patient care when they work together. This means that patients receive care that takes into account all aspects of their health, from physical to emotional and mental health.

Improved patient outcomes

Collaboration among healthcare providers has been shown to improve patient outcomes. This is because when providers work together, they can identify potential problems and address them before they become serious.

Increased efficiency

Collaboration among healthcare providers can also increase efficiency in the delivery of healthcare. By working together, providers can streamline care and reduce duplication of effort.

Enhanced communication

Collaborating with healthcare providers can enhance communication between different members of the care team. This means that everyone involved in a patient's care is aware of what is happening and can work together to ensure that the patient receives the best possible care.

Improved patient satisfaction

Patients who receive care from a team of healthcare providers are more likely to be satisfied with their care. This is because they receive comprehensive care that addresses needs and challenges holistically.

Prevention and early detection of health issues

Healthcare providers who collaborate can more effectively prevent and detect health issues. For example, a primary care doctor may notice symptoms that require further evaluation by a specialist, or a pharmacist may identify potential drug interactions that could cause harm. By working together, healthcare providers can ensure that patients receive the care they need at the earliest possible stage.

Improved use of resources

Collaboration among healthcare providers can ensure that resources are used more efficiently. For example, instead of ordering duplicate tests or procedures, providers can share information and work together to determine the best course of action for the patient.

Better coordination of care

Collaboration among healthcare providers can improve coordination of care for patients who have complex medical needs. For example, a patient with multiple chronic conditions may require care from several different specialists, and collaboration among those specialists can help to ensure that the patient's care is well coordinated and effective.

Enhanced patient education

Collaboration among healthcare providers can also enhance patient education. For example, a nurse may provide guidance on medication use, a physical therapist may provide information on exercises to improve mobility, and a nutritionist may provide advice on healthy eating. By working together, providers can ensure that patients receive a comprehensive education on how to manage their health.

Improved job satisfaction

Collaboration among healthcare providers can also improve job satisfaction. Providers who feel like they are part of a cohesive team are more likely to feel engaged in their work and more satisfied with their jobs. This can improve staff retention and create a more positive work environment.

In conclusion, collaboration with healthcare providers is essential for delivering high-quality healthcare. By working together, providers can improve patient outcomes, increase efficiency, enhance communication, prevent and detect health issues, improve resource use, coordinate care, enhance patient education, and improve job satisfaction.

B. How to Find a Healthcare Provider

who Supports Natural Healing

Finding a healthcare provider who supports natural healing depends on where your location and the type of healthcare provider you are looking for. Here are some steps that can help you find a provider who supports natural healing:

Research

Start by doing some research online. Look for healthcare providers who specialize in natural healing or have experience in complementary and alternative medicine (CAM). You can use search engines like Google or Bing to find such practitioners, or directories like the American Association of Naturopathic Physicians, the National Center for Complementary and Integrative Health, and the American Holistic Medical Association.

Referrals

Ask friends, family members, or coworkers if they know of any natural healing practitioners in your area. Personal referrals can be a valuable source of information.

Check credentials

Before you make an appointment with a healthcare provider, check their credentials. Look for licensed professionals who have received training in natural healing or have certification in CAM.

Consultation

Schedule a consultation with the healthcare provider to discuss your health concerns and ask about their approach to natural healing. This will help you determine if they are a good fit for you.

Reviews and ratings

Check online reviews and ratings of the healthcare provider you are considering. This will give you an idea of what others have experienced while working with them.

Insurance coverage

Check with your insurance company to see if they cover natural healing services. Some insurance companies have policies that cover some forms of CAM, such as chiropractic care or acupuncture.

Determine what type of natural healing you are interested in

Natural healing can encompass a range of practices, including herbal medicine, acupuncture, chiropractic care, massage therapy, and many others. Before you start your search, consider which types of natural healing you are most interested in.

Consider seeing a naturopathic doctor

Naturopathic doctors (NDs) are licensed healthcare professionals who are trained to use natural remedies to help patients achieve and maintain optimal health. They focus on treating the whole person rather than just the symptoms of a disease. They can guide one on natural remedies, nutrition, and lifestyle changes.

Look for holistic practitioners

A holistic practitioner is someone who takes a whole-body approach to health and wellness. They may use a combination of natural and conventional treatments to help patients achieve optimal health. Holistic practitioners can include naturopathic doctors, chiropractors, acupuncturists, and other types of healthcare providers.

Consider the location

Look for natural healing practitioners that are located near your home or work. This can make it easier to schedule appointments and reduce the amount of time and energy needed to get to your appointments.

Ask about the provider's experience

When you speak to a healthcare provider, ask about their experience in natural healing. Ask about the types of conditions they have treated. Enquire about the natural remedies they have used to help patients achieve optimal health.

Check for licensing and certification

Make sure that the healthcare provider you choose is licensed or certified in their field. This can help ensure that they have the proper training and experience to provide you with safe and effective natural healing treatments.

Remember, it is important to find a healthcare provider that you feel comfortable with, and that aligns with your beliefs and values. Take your time to research and find a provider who can provide you with the care and support you need to achieve optimal health.

C. Communicating Effectively with your Healthcare Provider

Communicating effectively with your healthcare provider is critical to ensuring that you receive the best care.

Here are some tips that can help you communicate effectively with your healthcare provider:

Be prepared: Before your appointment, make a list of the questions you want to ask your healthcare provider. Write down any symptoms you have been experiencing and any concerns you may have.

Be honest: Be honest with your healthcare provider about your medical history, any medications you are taking, and any lifestyle factors that may be affecting your health.

Ask questions: If you need help understanding something your healthcare provider is saying, feel free to ask for clarification. Ask about the potential risks and benefits of any treatment options.

Take notes: It can be helpful to take notes during your appointment so you can refer to them later.

Be specific: When describing your symptoms, be as specific as possible. Use descriptive words to explain the severity, location, and duration of your symptoms.

Be an active participant: Participate in the decision-making process and ask for clarification if you are not sure about the next steps.

Follow-up: If you have any questions after your appointment, do not hesitate to follow up with your healthcare provider.

Bring a family member or friend: It can be helpful to bring a trusted family member or friend to your appointment, especially if you are feeling anxious or have trouble remembering important details.

Be aware of cultural differences: If you have cultural or language differences with your healthcare provider, make sure to communicate this to them. This can help ensure that your healthcare provider understands your needs and can tailor their approach accordingly.

Be respectful: Remember to be respectful to your healthcare provider, even if you disagree with their advice or approach. Maintaining a positive relationship with your healthcare provider is crucial for your overall health and well-being.

Discuss cost: If you are concerned about the cost of your healthcare, be sure to discuss this with your provider. They can suggest lower-cost alternatives or help you find financial assistance programs.

Keep track of your medical history: Keeping track of your medical history, including previous diagnoses, surgeries, and medications, can help you provide information that is more accurate to your healthcare provider.

Be patient: Healthcare providers may be busy, and appointments may be rushed. Remember to be patient and respectful, even if you feel like you are not getting enough time to discuss your concerns.

By following these tips, you can ensure that you communicate effectively with your healthcare provider and receive the best possible care.

D. Understanding the Role of Conventional Medicine in Reversing Chronic Diseases

Conventional medicine, which is also known as Western or modern medicine, plays a vital role in the management and treatment of chronic diseases. Chronic diseases are conditions that persist over time, and a variety of factors, such as genetic predisposition, lifestyle choices, environmental factors, or a combination of these, can cause them.

In order to reverse chronic diseases, conventional medicine typically focuses on treating the underlying causes of the disease and managing symptoms. This can involve a combination of medications, lifestyle changes, and other interventions.

For example, in the case of type 2 diabetes, conventional medicine may involve medications to help regulate blood sugar levels, as well as lifestyle changes such as dietary modifications and increased physical activity. For heart disease, conventional medicine may involve medications to lower blood pressure or cholesterol, as well as lifestyle changes such as smoking cessation and increased exercise.

In addition, conventional medicine often uses a multidisciplinary approach to managing chronic diseases, involving a team of healthcare professionals such as doctors, pharmacists, nurses, nutritionists, and physical therapists.

Here are some points to consider:

Diagnosis: Conventional medicine relies on evidence-based scientific research and uses diagnostic tools such as blood tests, imaging scans, and biopsies to identify the underlying causes of chronic diseases. Accurate diagnosis is crucial to developing an effective treatment plan.

Medications: Conventional medicine often uses medications to manage and treat chronic diseases. These medications may help to control symptoms, slow disease progression, or even reverse the disease in some cases. However, medications can have side effects and may not be effective for everyone.

Surgery: For some chronic diseases, such as certain types of cancer, surgery may be necessary to remove tumors or other affected tissue. Conventional medicine has advanced surgical techniques to minimize the risk and improve outcomes for these procedures.

Prevention: Conventional medicine emphasizes the importance of preventing chronic diseases through lifestyle changes such as a healthy diet, regular exercise, stress reduction, and smoking cessation. Early detection through regular screening and check-ups can also help to prevent or manage chronic diseases.

Limitations: Conventional medicine may have only some of the answers when it comes to treating chronic diseases, and there may be cases where it could be more effective or suitable for a particular individual. In these cases, complementary or alternative approaches may be considered.

While conventional medicine can be highly effective in managing and even reversing some chronic diseases, it is instructive to note that it is not the only approach. Integrative or complementary medicine, which combines conventional and alternative medicine, is another approach that can be effective in managing chronic diseases. Ultimately, the best approach will depend on the individual's specific needs and preferences.

E. Integrating Natural and Alternative therapies with Conventional Medicine

Integrating natural and alternative therapies with conventional medicine can provide patients with a more comprehensive and holistic approach to their healthcare needs. Conventional medicine refers to the standard Western medical treatments, such as medications and surgeries. At the same time, natural and alternative therapies include non-traditional approaches to healing, such as acupuncture, massage, and herbal medicine.

Important considerations when integrating natural and alternative therapies with conventional medicine:

Ensure you consult with a healthcare professional

It is essential to consult with a qualified healthcare professional before starting any new therapies. They can help you determine which therapies may be helpful for your condition and ensure they are safe and appropriate for you.

Communication is key:

It is important to inform your healthcare provider about any natural or alternative therapies you are using. This can help prevent potential adverse interactions with any medications or treatments you are receiving.

Collaborative approach

Integrating natural and alternative therapies with conventional medicine should be done collaboratively. Healthcare providers from different fields should work together to develop a comprehensive treatment plan that addresses the patient's needs.

Evidence-based approach

When considering natural and alternative therapies, it is important to look for evidence-based practices. This means that there is scientific evidence to support their effectiveness and safety.

Patient-centered approach

It is crucial to prioritize the patient's goals and preferences when developing a treatment plan. Patients should be empowered to make informed decisions about their healthcare and have the option to choose therapies that align with their values and beliefs.

Quality control

Ensure that any natural or alternative therapies you use are of high quality and come from reputable sources. This can help minimize the risk of contamination or adulteration.

Safety considerations

Be aware of potential side effects or risks associated with natural and alternative therapies. Some may interact with conventional medications, and others may not be appropriate for specific medical conditions. Always consult with a qualified healthcare professional to ensure that any therapies you use are safe and appropriate for you.

Mind-body techniques

In addition to physical therapies, mind-body techniques such as meditation, yoga, and mindfulness can be effective in managing stress, anxiety, and pain. These techniques can complement conventional treatments and improve overall well-being.

Integrative medicine specialists

Consider seeking out an integrative medicine specialist or center that offers a range of natural and alternative therapies in conjunction with conventional medicine. These specialists can help develop a personalized treatment plan that meets your unique healthcare needs.

Education and self-care

In addition to receiving therapies, patients can also benefit from education and self-care practices that promote health and well-being. This includes things like healthy eating, regular exercise, and stress management techniques. Empowering patients to take an active role in their health can help improve treatment outcomes and overall quality of life. Integrating natural and alternative therapies with conventional medicine can be a valuable approach to healthcare. Still, it is necessary to approach it in a responsible and informed manner. By working with qualified healthcare professionals and prioritizing patient-centered care, patients can achieve better health outcomes and improve their overall well-being.

VI: PUTTING IT ALL TOGETHER

A. Developing a Personalized Plan for Reversing Chronic Diseases

Developing a personalized plan for reversing chronic diseases can be a complex process that requires a multidisciplinary approach. Here are some general steps that can be taken to develop such a plan:

Consult with a healthcare professional

The first step in developing a personalized plan for reversing chronic diseases is to consult with a healthcare professional, such as a doctor, pharmacist, nurse, or registered dietitian. They can provide an assessment of your current health status, identify any risk factors, and develop a plan based on your specific needs.

Identify the underlying cause

It is essential to identify the underlying cause of your chronic disease, whether it is related to diet, lifestyle, genetics, or environmental factors. This can help guide in the development of a personalized plan that addresses the root cause of the problem.

Medication review

Your pharmacist will review all your medication to rule out any drug-drug or drug-food interactions.

Develop a nutrition plan

Nutrition is a critical component of any plan for reversing chronic diseases. A registered dietitian can develop a personalized nutrition plan that takes into account your specific health needs and dietary restrictions. The plan should emphasize whole foods, fruits & vegetables, lean protein, and healthy fats while limiting processed foods, sugary beverages, and excess salt.

Develop an exercise plan

Exercise is also a critical component of any plan for reversing chronic diseases. A healthcare professional can help develop an exercise plan that takes into account your current fitness level, medical history, and any physical limitations. The plan should include both aerobic and strength training exercises and aim for at least 30 minutes of moderate activity most days of the week.

Address lifestyle factors

Lifestyle factors such as stress, sleep, and smoking can also play a role in chronic diseases. Developing healthy habits around these factors can improve overall health and reduce the risk of chronic diseases. For example, developing a stress management plan, getting adequate sleep, and quitting smoking can all have significant impacts on health.

Monitor progress

It is essential to monitor progress regularly to determine whether the personalized plan is effective in reversing the chronic disease. This can be done through regular check-ins with a healthcare professional, tracking of symptoms, and monitoring of key health metrics such as blood pressure, cholesterol, and blood sugar levels.

Identify potential barriers and develop strategies to overcome them

There may be barriers that could hinder progress in reversing chronic diseases, such as lack of time, financial constraints, or social support. It is important to identify these barriers and develop strategies to overcome them. For example, finding affordable healthy food options or incorporating physical activity into daily routines can help overcome these challenges.

Consider complementary and alternative therapies

In addition to conventional medical treatments, many complementary and alternative therapies may be beneficial for chronic diseases, such as acupuncture, massage therapy, and herbal medicine. It is essential to work with a healthcare professional to determine which therapies may be appropriate and safe.

Engage in community support

Joining a community or support group can provide motivation, accountability, and emotional support when making lifestyle changes. Local resources such as community centers or online support groups can help individuals connect with others who are working towards similar goals.

Maintain a positive mindset

Reversing chronic diseases can be a long and challenging process, and maintaining a positive mindset is essential for success. Celebrating small successes, focusing on progress rather than perfection and practicing self-compassion can help individuals stay motivated and engaged in their health journey.

Developing a personalized plan for reversing chronic diseases requires a comprehensive approach that takes into account individual needs, risk factors, and barriers. Working with a healthcare professional and incorporating healthy lifestyle habits, complementary therapies, community support, and a positive mindset can help individuals achieve their health goals and improve their overall quality of life.

B. Implementing Lifestyle Changes and Natural Therapies

Implementing lifestyle changes and natural therapies can have a positive impact on overall health and well-being. Here are some suggestions:

Diet: Eating a healthy and balanced diet is essential for good health. Include plenty of fruits and vegetables, lean proteins, whole grains, and healthy fats in your diet. Avoid processed foods, sugary drinks, and excessive amounts of alcohol.

Exercise: Regular physical activity can improve overall health and well-being. Try to engage in at least 30 minutes of moderate-intensity exercise most days of the week. You can try walking, jogging, swimming, or any other activity that you enjoy.

Stress management: Stress can negatively affect health. Practice stress management techniques such as meditation, deep breathing, yoga, or tai chi to help reduce stress levels.

Sleep: Adequate sleep is essential for good health. Try to get 7-8 hours of sleep each night and establish a consistent sleep routine.

Natural therapies: Consider incorporating natural therapies such as acupuncture, massage, herbal remedies, or aromatherapy into your healthcare routine. These can help alleviate symptoms and improve overall well-being.

Hydration: Drinking enough water is essential for overall health. Aim to drink at least eight glasses of water each day and more if you are physically active or in hot weather.

Mindfulness: Practicing mindfulness can help reduce stress and improve overall well-being. Try incorporating techniques like mindful breathing, visualization, or body scans into your daily routine.

Sunlight and fresh air: Spending time outside can help boost mood and energy levels. Aim to spend at least 30 minutes outside each day, especially during daylight hours.

Social connections: Having strong social connections can improve mental health and well-being. Try to regularly connect with friends and family, join a club or group, or volunteer in your community.

Supplements: Certain supplements may have beneficial effects on overall health. Talk to your healthcare professional about which supplements may be right for you.

Remember, making small changes over time can lead to significant improvements in overall health and well-being. Start by incorporating one or two of these lifestyle changes or natural therapies and gradually build from there. It is also important to be patient and kind to yourself throughout the process.

C. Monitoring Progress and Making Adjustments

When it comes to reversing chronic diseases, monitoring progress and making adjustments are essential steps to ensure success. Here are some strategies for doing so:

Tracking Progress: Regular monitoring of the disease and its related symptoms can help to gauge the success of the treatment. This can include regular check-ups with a doctor or specialist, monitoring blood pressure, blood sugar levels, or other relevant indicators.

Setting Goals: Setting achievable goals helps keep the patient motivated and focused on their progress. These goals should be specific, measurable, and achievable within a reasonable timeframe.

Adjusting Treatment: Treatment plans may need to be adjusted as the disease progresses or if the patient is not responding to treatment. This may involve changes to medication, lifestyle modifications, or other interventions.

Patient Education: Providing patients with education and resources can help them understand their condition and the steps they can take to manage it. This may include information on nutrition, exercise, stress management, and other lifestyle factors that can impact their disease.

Supportive Care: Supportive care can help to improve the patient's overall well-being and quality of life. This may include access to counseling, support groups, or other resources to help manage the emotional and psychological impact of the disease.

Utilize Technology: There are numerous apps and wearable devices that can help patients track their progress in real time. For example, a patient with diabetes can use a glucose-monitoring app to track their blood sugar levels throughout the day.

Engage in Self-Monitoring: Patients can also take an active role in monitoring their condition by self-monitoring. This may include keeping a food diary, tracking physical activity, or monitoring symptoms.

Regularly Review Treatment Plans: Review treatment plans regularly to ensure they are still effective and appropriate. This can be done in collaboration with the patient's healthcare team.

Encourage Compliance: Compliance with treatment is essential for achieving positive outcomes. Healthcare providers should work with patients to identify barriers to compliance and develop strategies to overcome them.

Address Comorbidities: Patients with chronic diseases often have other health conditions that can affect their overall health. Healthcare providers should address any comorbidity and develop a comprehensive treatment plan that addresses all of the patient's health needs.

By utilizing these strategies, patients and healthcare providers can work together to effectively monitor progress and make adjustments in reversing chronic diseases. This can lead to better health outcomes, improved quality of life, and reduced healthcare costs over time.

D. Maintaining Good Health and Preventing Chronic Diseases in the Future

Maintaining good health and preventing chronic diseases involves a combination of healthy lifestyle choices and regular medical check-ups. Here are some steps you can take to maintain good health:

Eat a healthy diet: A healthy diet includes a variety of fruits, vegetables, whole grains, lean proteins, and healthy fats. Avoid processed and junk food as much as possible.

Exercise regularly: Physical activity is crucial for maintaining good health. Aim for at least 30 minutes of moderate-intensity exercise, such as brisk walking, cycling, or swimming, most days of the week.

Maintain a healthy weight: Obesity is a risk factor for many chronic diseases, including diabetes, heart disease, and cancer. To maintain a healthy weight, eat a balanced diet and exercise regularly.

Get enough sleep: Lack of sleep can increase the risk of chronic diseases, such as obesity, diabetes, and depression. Aim for at least seven hours of sleep per night.

Manage stress: Chronic stress can lead to a host of health problems, including high blood pressure, heart disease, and depression. Find ways to manage stress, such as meditation, yoga, or deep breathing exercises.

Limit alcohol intake: Drinking too much alcohol can increase the risk of liver disease, cancer, and other health problems. If you choose to drink, do so in moderation.

Avoid smoking and secondhand smoke: Smoking and exposure to secondhand smoke increase the risk of lung cancer, heart disease, stroke, and other health problems. Quit smoking if you currently smoke and avoid exposure to secondhand smoke as much as possible.

Get regular check-ups: Regular check-ups can help detect health problems early when they are easier to treat. Make sure to schedule regular appointments with your healthcare provider, including screenings for chronic diseases such as diabetes, high blood pressure, and cancer.

Practice good hygiene: Regular hand washing, brushing and flossing your teeth, and practicing safe sex, are all important steps in maintaining good health and preventing the spread of disease.

Protect yourself from the sun: Exposure to the sun's harmful UV rays can increase the risk of skin cancer. Protect yourself by wearing sunscreen with a high SPF, covering exposed skin with clothing, and avoiding prolonged exposure to the sun, especially during peak hours.

Stay hydrated: Drinking enough water is essential for maintaining good health. Aim for at least 8-10 glasses of water per day, more if you are physically active or live in a hot climate.

Stay up-to-date on vaccinations: Vaccines are an important way to prevent many serious illnesses, including the flu, pneumonia, and certain types of cancer. Make sure you are up-to-date on all recommended vaccinations.

Practice safe behaviors: Avoid risky behaviors, such as driving under the influence of alcohol, texting while driving, and not wearing a seatbelt. These behaviors can increase the risk of severe injury to death.

Stay socially connected: Maintaining social connections is important for good mental health and overall well-being. Make an effort to stay connected with family and friends, join a social group, or volunteer in your community.

Be proactive with your health: Take an active role in your health by learning about your family's medical history, understanding your risk factors for chronic diseases, and asking your healthcare provider questions about your health.

By incorporating these steps into your daily routine, you can reduce your risk of chronic diseases and maintain good health for years to come.

E. Importance of a Supportive Community and Finding One

A supportive community can play a crucial role in helping individuals reverse chronic diseases. Chronic diseases, such as diabetes, heart disease, and obesity, can be challenging to manage and often require significant lifestyle changes, such as adopting a healthy diet and increasing physical activity. A supportive community can provide individuals with the motivation, encouragement, and accountability needed to make these changes and stick to them.

Ways to find a supportive community in reversing chronic diseases:

Join a support group: There are many support groups for individuals with chronic diseases. These groups can provide a safe and supportive environment for individuals to share their experiences, learn from others, and receive emotional support.

Attend community events: Many communities offer events and activities focused on healthy living, such as cooking classes, fitness classes, and health fairs. Attending these events can help individuals connect with like-minded people who are also interested in reversing chronic diseases.

Find an workout buddy: Finding a friend or family member who shares the same health goals can provide a source of motivation and accountability for individuals trying to reverse chronic diseases. Exercising together can also make the experience more enjoyable.

Seek professional support: Working with a healthcare professional, such as a registered dietitian, a personal trainer, or a therapist, can provide individuals with the guidance and support they need to manage their chronic disease effectively. These professionals can also connect individuals with local resources and support groups.

Use social media: Social media platforms such as Facebook and Instagram can be great places to find supportive communities of individuals with similar health goals. There are many groups and pages dedicated to topics like healthy eating, fitness, and disease management. Joining these groups can provide individuals with a source of inspiration and motivation, as well as a space to ask questions and share experiences.

Volunteer: Volunteering with organizations focused on health and wellness can be a great way to connect with others who share similar interests and goals. Volunteering provides individuals with a sense of purpose and fulfillment, which is essential for maintaining motivation and engagement in the process of reversing chronic diseases.

Attend workshops and seminars: Many organizations and healthcare facilities offer workshops and seminars focused on chronic disease management and prevention. Attending these events can provide individuals with the opportunity to learn from experts, connect with others who are on a similar journey, and gain new insights and strategies for managing their chronic disease.

Join an online community: In addition to social media, there are many online communities and forums focused on chronic disease management and prevention. These communities can provide individuals with a space to connect with others who understand the challenges of living with a chronic disease, share resources and information, and receive support and encouragement.

Finding a supportive community is crucial for individuals trying to reverse chronic diseases. Whether it is through joining a support group, attending community events, finding an exercise buddy, seeking professional support, using social media, volunteering, attending workshops and seminars, or joining an online community, there are many ways to connect with others who can provide the support, encouragement, and accountability needed to achieve health goals and improve quality of life.

VII:CASE STUDIES AND SUCCESS STORIES

A. Real-Life Examples of Individuals
Who Have Reversed Chronic Diseases

There are many real-life examples of people who have successfully reversed chronic diseases through lifestyle changes and other interventions. Here are a few examples:

1. Dean Ornish

Dr. Dean Ornish is a renowned physician and researcher who developed the Ornish Lifestyle Medicine program, which emphasizes a low-fat, plant-based diet, stress reduction techniques, exercise, and social support. His program has been shown to reverse heart disease, type 2 diabetes, and other chronic diseases.

2. Dr. Terry Wahls

Dr. Terry Wahls is a physician who reversed her multiple sclerosis (MS) through diet and lifestyle changes. She developed the Wahls Protocol, which involves a nutrient-dense diet, exercise, and other interventions. Her protocol has been shown to improve symptoms in people with MS and other autoimmune conditions.

3. Dr. Caldwell Esselstyn

Dr. Caldwell Esselstyn is a physician and researcher who developed the Plant-Based Nutrition Program at the Cleveland Clinic. His program emphasizes a low-fat, plant-based diet and has been shown to reverse heart disease in many patients.

4. Jason Fung

Dr. Jason Fung is a nephrologist who has helped many patients reverse type 2 diabetes through a low-carbohydrate, high-fat diet and intermittent fasting.

5. Dr. Michael Greger

Dr. Michael Greger is a physician and founder of NutritionFacts.org. This website provides evidence-based information on nutrition and health. He has helped many patients reverse chronic diseases through a plant-based diet and other interventions.

6. Dr. Joel Fuhrman

Dr. Joel Fuhrman is a physician and author who advocates for a plant-based, nutrient-dense diet to reverse chronic diseases. He has helped many patients reverse type 2 diabetes, heart disease, and other chronic conditions through diet and lifestyle changes.

7. Dr. John McDougall

Dr. John McDougall is a physician and author who advocates for a low-fat, plant-based diet to reverse chronic diseases. His program has been shown to reverse heart disease, type 2 diabetes, and other chronic conditions.

8. Dr. Neal Barnard

Dr. Neal Barnard is a physician and author who advocates for a plant-based diet to reverse chronic diseases. His program has been shown to reverse type 2 diabetes, heart disease, and other chronic conditions.

9. Sami Inkinen

Sami Inkinen is a technology entrepreneur and triathlete who reversed his insulin resistance and type 2 diabetes through a low-carbohydrate, high-fat diet and exercise. He has since founded a company, Virta Health, which provides remote coaching and medical care to help people reverse type 2 diabetes.

10. Dr. Brooke Goldner

Dr. Brooke Goldner is a physician who reversed her lupus through a plant-based diet and other interventions. She has since helped many patients reverse autoimmune diseases through her Goodbye Lupus program.

These are just a few examples of people who have successfully reversed chronic diseases through diet and lifestyle changes. It is important to note that everyone's journey to better health is unique, and what works for one person may not work for another. Consulting with a qualified healthcare provider is essential when implementing any changes to your diet or medical treatment.

B. Lessons Learned from These Success Stories

There are many success stories of people who have reversed chronic diseases through lifestyle changes, such as changes to their diet, exercise routine, and stress management techniques. Some of the key lessons we can learn from these stories include:

The power of lifestyle changes

Many chronic diseases are preventable and even reversible through lifestyle changes. By adopting healthy habits like regular exercise, a nutritious diet, and stress management techniques, people can improve their overall health and potentially reverse chronic conditions.

Personalized approach

There is no one-size-fits-all solution to reversing chronic diseases.

Each person's body and health condition is unique, and what works for one person may not work for another. It is essential to work with a healthcare professional to develop a personalized plan for your health.

Consistency is Key

Consistency is crucial when it comes to making lifestyle changes that can reverse chronic diseases. Making small, sustainable changes to your daily routine over time can help you build healthy habits that last.

Mind-body connection

The mind-body connection is a critical component of overall health. Incorporating practices like meditation, yoga, and other relaxation techniques can help reduce stress and promote healing.

The importance of community

Having a supportive community can be incredibly beneficial when making lifestyle changes to reverse chronic diseases. Connecting with others who share similar health goals can provide motivation and accountability.

Importance of education and knowledge

Many people who have successfully reversed chronic diseases have emphasized the importance of education and knowledge. Understanding how certain foods and lifestyle factors impact health can help people make informed choices and take control of their health.

Addressing root causes

Addressing the underlying causes of chronic diseases is crucial in reversing them. This may involve identifying and addressing nutritional deficiencies, addressing chronic stress, or identifying and removing environmental toxins.

Patience and persistence

Reversing chronic diseases is not an overnight process. It takes time, patience, and persistence to make lasting lifestyle changes and see significant improvements in health.

Positive mindset

A positive mindset can make a significant difference in the journey of reversing chronic diseases. Believing in one's ability to make positive changes and focusing on progress rather than perfection can help people stay motivated and committed to their goals.

Holistic approach

Taking a holistic approach to health can be beneficial when reversing chronic diseases. This involves addressing physical, mental, and emotional health and may involve incorporating practices like acupuncture, massage therapy, or other complementary therapies alongside lifestyle changes.

These lessons demonstrate that reversing chronic diseases requires a multifaceted approach that addresses both physical and mental health, involves education and knowledge, and emphasizes patience, persistence, and a positive mindset. By taking a holistic approach, people can improve their overall health and potentially reverse chronic conditions.

VIII:CONCLUSION

A. Summary of Key Points

Reversing chronic diseases is possible by making specific lifestyle changes and seeking medical treatment, depending on the type and severity of the condition. Here are some key points:

1. Change your diet: Consuming a healthy diet consisting of fruits, vegetables, whole grains, and lean protein sources can help prevent and even reverse chronic diseases.

2. Exercise regularly: Regular exercise can help improve heart health, control blood sugar levels, and reduce inflammation, all of which can help prevent and reverse chronic diseases.

3. Quit smoking: Smoking is a significant risk factor for many chronic diseases, and quitting smoking can help reduce the risk of developing these conditions and may even help reverse some of the damage caused by smoking.

4. Manage stress: Chronic stress can contribute to the development and progression of chronic diseases. Therefore, practicing stress-reducing techniques like meditation, yoga, and deep breathing can be helpful.

5. Get enough sleep: Adequate sleep is essential for overall health and can help reduce the risk of developing chronic diseases.

6. Seek medical treatment: Depending on the type and severity of the chronic disease, medical treatment may be necessary. This may include medications, surgery, or other medical procedures.

7. Follow medical advice: It is essential to follow medical advice, take medications as prescribed, and attend follow-up appointments with healthcare providers to manage chronic diseases effectively.

8. Make lifestyle changes: Making lifestyle changes can be challenging, but it is essential for preventing and reversing chronic diseases. It may require support from family, friends, and healthcare providers to make these changes successfully.

9. Maintain a healthy weight: Being overweight or obese is a significant risk factor for many chronic diseases, including diabetes, heart disease, and certain types of cancer. Losing weight through a combination of healthy eating and exercise can help prevent and reverse these conditions.

10. Control blood sugar levels: High blood sugar levels can lead to diabetes and other chronic conditions. By controlling blood sugar levels through a healthy diet, exercise, and medication, you can help prevent and reverse these conditions.

11. Lower cholesterol levels: High cholesterol levels can contribute to the development of heart disease and other chronic conditions. Eating a healthy diet, exercising regularly, and taking medication as prescribed can help lower cholesterol levels and reduce the risk of these conditions.

12. Manage high blood pressure: High blood pressure is a risk factor for heart disease, stroke, and other chronic conditions. Eating a healthy diet, exercising regularly, and taking medication as prescribed can help manage high blood pressure and reduce the risk of these conditions.

13. Reduce inflammation: Chronic inflammation is associated with many chronic diseases, including arthritis, heart disease, and diabetes. Eating a healthy diet that includes anti-inflammatory foods like fruits, vegetables, and whole grains and avoiding pro-inflammatory foods like processed and fried foods can help reduce inflammation.

14. Limit alcohol consumption: Drinking too much alcohol can increase the risk of developing chronic diseases like liver disease, heart disease, and cancer. Limiting alcohol consumption to moderate levels or avoiding it altogether can help prevent and reverse these conditions.

15. Address mental health: Chronic diseases can take a toll on mental health, and vice versa. Addressing mental health through therapy, medication, or other treatments can help manage chronic diseases and improve overall health and well-being.

16. Stay up-to-date with screenings and check-ups: Regular screenings and check-ups can help detect chronic diseases early when they are more manageable and treatable. Be sure to stay up-to-date with recommended screenings and check-ups for your age and gender.

B. Final Thoughts and Encouragement

Reversing chronic diseases can be a challenging journey, but it is also an incredibly worthwhile and life-changing one. With commitment, patience, and support, it is possible to achieve significant improvements in your health and quality of life.

Some final thoughts and encouragement for reversing chronic diseases:

Believe in yourself: The power of the mind is incredible, and having a positive attitude can make all the difference in your journey towards reversing chronic diseases. Believe that you can achieve your health goals and stay motivated and focused on your progress.

Seek support: You do not have to go through this journey alone. Seek support from family, friends, or a healthcare professional. Joining a support group or finding an accountability partner can also be helpful in staying motivated and on track.

Educate yourself: Learn as much as you can about your condition and the lifestyle changes that can help reverse it. This knowledge can empower you to make informed decisions about your health and create a personalized plan that works for you.

Start small: Making significant lifestyle changes can be overwhelming, so start small and gradually build up to changes that are more considerable. Focus on making one change at a time, whether it is increasing physical activity or improving your diet.

Celebrate your successes: Celebrate every small success along the way. Reversing chronic diseases is a journey, and progress can take time. Acknowledge and celebrate your efforts and progress, no matter how small they may seem.

Focus on whole, nutrient-dense foods: One of the most effective ways to reverse chronic diseases is by focusing on whole, nutrient-dense foods. These foods are rich in vitamins, minerals, and antioxidants, which can help reduce inflammation, improve insulin sensitivity, and promote overall health. Incorporate plenty of fresh fruits and vegetables, lean protein sources, whole grains, and healthy fats into your diet.

Move your body: Regular physical activity is crucial for reversing chronic diseases. Exercise can help improve cardiovascular health, lower blood pressure, improve insulin sensitivity, and reduce inflammation. Start with small steps, like taking a walk around the block, and gradually increase the intensity and duration of your workouts.

Practice stress management: Chronic stress can contribute to a range of health issues, including cardiovascular disease, diabetes, and depression. Incorporate stress-reducing activities into your routine, such as meditation, yoga, deep breathing exercises, or spending time in nature.

Get enough sleep: Getting enough sleep is essential for overall health and can help reduce inflammation, improve insulin sensitivity, and support healthy immune function. Aim for seven to eight hours of sleep per night, and establish a consistent sleep routine.

Do not give up: Reversing chronic diseases is a journey that can be filled with setbacks and challenges. Remember that progress takes time, and setbacks are a natural part of the process. Do not give up, even if you experience setbacks. Instead, use them as an opportunity to learn and adjust your approach.

In conclusion, reversing chronic diseases requires dedication, patience, and a commitment to making healthy lifestyle changes. By focusing on whole, nutrient-dense foods, regular physical activity, stress management, and quality sleep, you can achieve significant improvements in your health and well-being. Remember to stay positive, seek support, and celebrate your successes along the way.

C. Additional Resources for Reversing Chronic Diseases

Reversing chronic diseases often requires a multifaceted approach that involves lifestyle changes, dietary modifications, and medical interventions. Here are some resources that can help you in your journey to reverse chronic diseases:

1. **The Centers for Disease Control and Prevention (CDC)** has a wealth of information on chronic disease prevention and management. Their website offers a variety of resources on topics such as healthy eating, physical activity, and disease management.

2. The American Heart Association (AHA) provides information and resources on heart disease prevention and management. They offer tips on healthy eating, physical activity, and stress. The American Diabetes Association (ADA) provides resources for people with diabetes, including management.

3. Information on managing blood sugar levels, healthy eating, and physical activity.

4. The National Institute of Diabetes and Digestive and Kidney Diseases (NIDDK) offers resources on diabetes prevention and management, as well as other digestive and kidney diseases.

5. **The Arthritis Foundation** provides resources for people with arthritis, including information on managing pain, staying active and healthy eating.

6. The National Cancer Institute provides information on cancer prevention and management, including resources on healthy eating, physical activity, and screening.

7. The American Lung Association provides information on lung health and disease management, including resources on quitting smoking, managing asthma, and coping with chronic lung disease.

8. The Mayo Clinic offers information on a wide range of health topics, including chronic disease prevention and management. Their website offers articles, videos, and other resources on healthy living, disease management, and medical treatments.

9. The Harvard Medical School offers a variety of health-related resources, including articles on chronic disease prevention and management. Their website also offers information on medical treatments, clinical trials, and research.

10. The Cleveland Clinic provides information on a variety of health topics, including chronic disease prevention and management. Their website offers articles, videos, and other resources on healthy living, disease management, and medical treatments.

11. World Health Organization (WHO) - The WHO provides a wide range of resources on chronic disease prevention and management, including information on healthy lifestyles, risk factors, and medical treatments. The WHO also offers guidance on developing policies and strategies for chronic disease prevention and management at the national level.

12. African Diabetes Alliance - The African Diabetes Alliance is a non-profit organization that aims to improve diabetes prevention and management in Africa. They offer resources for patients, healthcare professionals, and policymakers, including information on healthy lifestyles, medical treatments, and policy development.

13. African Heart Network - The African Heart Network is a non-profit organization that focuses on cardiovascular disease prevention and management in Africa. They offer resources for patients, healthcare professionals, and policymakers, including information on healthy lifestyles, medical treatments, and policy development.

14. Diabetes South Africa - Diabetes South Africa is a non-profit organization that provides resources for diabetes prevention and management in South Africa. They offer information on healthy eating, physical activity, and medical treatments, as well as support groups and other resources for patients.

15. Diabetes Ghana - Diabetes Ghana is a non-profit organization that provides resources for diabetes prevention and management in Ghana. They offer information on healthy eating, physical activity, and medical treatments, as well as support groups and other resources for patients.

16. Nigerian Heart Foundation - The Nigerian Heart Foundation is a non-profit organization that focuses on cardiovascular disease prevention and management in Nigeria. They offer resources for patients, healthcare professionals, and policymakers, including information on healthy lifestyles, medical treatments, and policy development.

17. The Heart and Stroke Foundation South Africa - The Heart and Stroke Foundation South Africa is a non-profit organization that focuses on cardiovascular disease prevention and management in South Africa. They offer resources for patients, healthcare professionals, and policymakers, including information on healthy lifestyles, medical treatments, and policy development.

18. The Chronic Disease Initiative for Africa - The Chronic Disease Initiative for Africa is a non-profit organization that focuses on chronic disease prevention and management in Africa. They offer resources for patients, healthcare professionals, and policymakers, including information on healthy lifestyles, medical treatments, and policy development.

It is important to note that these resources are not a substitute for medical advice. Always consult with a healthcare professional before making changes to your diet, exercise routine, or medical treatment plan.

D. The Future of Reversing Chronic Diseases and the Impact on Public Health

The future of reversing chronic diseases is promising as advancements in medical research and technology continue to evolve. Chronic diseases, such as heart disease, cancer, and diabetes, are responsible for a significant portion of deaths worldwide and reversing or managing these diseases could have a significant impact on public health.

One of the most significant advancements in the treatment of chronic diseases is the use of personalized medicine. This approach takes into account an individual's genetics, lifestyle, and environment to create a targeted treatment plan. By tailoring treatment plans to individual patients, healthcare providers can provide more effective and efficient care.

Another area of research that shows promise in reversing chronic diseases is regenerative medicine. This approach involves using stem cells or other methods to regenerate damaged tissues and organs. For example, researchers are exploring the use of stem cells to regenerate damaged heart tissue in patients with heart disease.

Additionally, lifestyle modifications such as diet and exercise can play a significant role in managing and even reversing chronic diseases. In recent years, there has been a growing body of research on the benefits of plant-based diets and exercise in preventing and reversing chronic diseases.

Other points to consider include:

1. **Early Detection and Prevention:** Early detection and prevention are key components in reversing chronic diseases. With advancements in medical technology, it is now possible to detect certain chronic diseases, such as cancer, at earlier stages when treatment is more effective. Additionally, lifestyle interventions such as regular exercise, maintaining a healthy weight, and avoiding tobacco use can prevent or delay the onset of many chronic diseases.

2. **Digital Health:** Digital health tools, such as wearable devices and mobile apps, are also playing an increasing role in managing and reversing chronic diseases. These tools can help patients monitor their symptoms, track their progress, and receive personalized recommendations for managing their condition.

3. **Health Equity:** One of the challenges in reversing chronic diseases is ensuring that all patients have access to the latest treatments and technologies. Health equity, which is the concept of ensuring that everyone has access to high-quality healthcare

regardless of their race, ethnicity, or socioeconomic status, is crucial in ensuring that all members of society feel the benefits of reversing chronic diseases.

4. Collaboration: Reversing chronic diseases will require collaboration between healthcare providers, researchers, policymakers, and patients. By working together, these groups can develop more effective treatment plans, improve access to care, and promote public health initiatives that reduce the risk of chronic diseases.

In conclusion, reversing chronic diseases is an important goal that has the potential to improve public health significantly. Advances in personalized medicine, regenerative medicine, lifestyle interventions, digital health, and health equity, along with collaboration between various stakeholders, offer promising pathways toward achieving this goal.

REFERENCES

Aggarwal, B. B., Van Kuiken, M. E., Iyer, L. H., & Harikumar, K. B. (2009). Molecular targets of nutraceuticals derived from dietary spices: potential role in suppression of inflammation and tumorigenesis. Experimental Biology and Medicine, 234(8), 825-849.

American College of Lifestyle Medicine. (2021). Lifestyle Medicine: The Evidence. https://www.lifestylemedicine.org/TheEvidence

American Heart Association. (2021). How much physical activity do you need? https://www.heart.org/en/healthy-living/fitness/fitness-basics/aha-recs-for- physical-activity-in-adults

American Holistic Medical Association. (2021). Find a Holistic Provider. https://www.holisticmedicine.org/find-a-provider/

Chopra, D. (2010). Reinventing the Body, Resurrecting the Soul: How to Create a New You. Harmony.

Centers for Disease Control and Prevention. (2021). Chronic Diseases in America. https://www.cdc.gov/chronic disease/resources/infographic/chronic-diseases.htm

Centers for Disease Control and Prevention. (2021). Preventing Chronic Disease: Public Health Research, Practice, and Policy. https://www.cdc.gov/pcd/ index.htm

Cohen, S., Kamarck, T., & Mermelstein, R. (1983). A Global Measure of Perceived Stress. Journal of Health and Social Behavior, 24(4), 385-396.

Environmental Protection Agency. (2021). Air Quality Index (AQI). https://www.epa.gov/air-quality-index

Esch, T., Fricchione, G. L., & Stefano, G. B. (2003). The therapeutic use of the relaxation response in stress-related diseases. Medical

Science Monitor, 9(2), RA23-34.

Greger, M. (2015). How Not to Die: Discover the Foods Scientifically Proven to Prevent and Reverse Disease. Flatiron Books.

Harvard Health Publishing. (2021). 10 diet changes to help reduce chronic pain. https://www.health.harvard.edu/pain/10-diet-changes-to-help-reduce-chronic-pain

Harvard Health Publishing. (2021). How to make lifestyle changes that last. https://www.health.harvard.edu/staying-healthy/how-to-make- lifestyle-changes-that-last

Higginbotham, E. J., & Taube, C. (2019). Chronic Diseases: An Encyclopedia of Causes, Effects, and Treatments. ABC-CLIO.

National Sleep Foundation. (2021). How Much Sleep Do We Really Need? https://www.sleepfoundation.org/how-sleep-works/how-much-sleep-do-we-really-need

National Center for Complementary and Integrative Health. (2021). Herbs at a Glance

National Center for Complementary and Integrative Health. (2021). Integrative Medicine: What You Need To Know. https://www.nccih.nih.gov/health/integrative- medicine

National Center for Complementary and Integrative Health. (2021). Talking With Your Health Care Providers About Complementary Health Approaches. https://www.nccih.nih.gov/health/tips/talking-with-your-health-care-providers-about-complementary-health-approaches

Ornish, D. (1998). Eat More, Weigh Less: Dr. Dean Ornish's Life Choice Program for Losing Weight Safely While Eating Abundantly. Harper Collins.

Ornish, D., Scherwitz, L. W., Billings, J. H., Brown, S. E., Gould, K. L., Merritt, T. A., ... & Brand, R. J. (1998). Intensive lifestyle changes for reversal of coronary heart disease. JAMA, 280(23), 2001-2007.

Willett, W. C. (2012). Eat, Drink, and Be Healthy: The Harvard Medical School Guide to Healthy Eating. Simon and Schuster.

World Health Organization. (2013). Global Action Plan for

the Prevention and Control of Non-communicable Diseases 2013-2020.
https://www.who.int/publications/i/item/9789241506236

World Health Organization. (2018). Noncommunicable Diseases. https://www.who.int/news-room/fact-sheets/detail/noncommunicable-diseases

World Health Organization. (2019). Chronic diseases and health promotion. https://www.who.int/chp/about/integrated_cd/en/